Pincushion

Contents

Foreword

I sat by her side, not sure how she was going to make it back to normal life for a woman in her early twenties.

'It writes things. It's like a pencil,' I watched her struggle to find the right words for the name of a simple ball point pen.

'It doesn't have lead but it has ink,' she said, with frustration, almost as if to convince herself and God to come to an agreement that she would be allowed to make this next step in recovery, begging for success.

She reached through the tub of dry rice and pulled out a pen, a rubber ball and a single dice. She shook with frustration as the rice irritated her skin; after all she was regaining feeling and mobility in her left side. Her brain haemorrhage and resulting stroke had caused both physical and cognitive disconnects, and maybe she could walk again. I held back my tears, and the rehabilitation specialist and I shared a knowing look. It was clear that she was trying her best. That day, I saw the beauty that God held as a secret from all of us, only for her to be, and me to have. She is stronger than any person I have ever met, and more beautiful than anything or anyone that I have ever seen.

Prepping for surgery is always a system. I pack the same things every time, call her Mom, and be the man God made me to be. I always cry in front of her, but come surgery time, I still cry, but at strategic times.

'Dear, you forgot your blanket,' I said as we walked towards the car.

She had a tired and beautiful blanket that was created for her as a young girl, many patches from various times. She had it with her for every one of her umpteen surgeries to date.

She paused, looked at me, smiled, and with her huge, uneven pupils looked at me, 'I don't need my blanket; I have you from now on.'

Her name is Elise and she is my wife.

Love, Aaron.

Introduction

Idiopathic, Intracranial, and Hypertension were once just words. An assortment of syllables with no meaning to me.

Countless words make up a person. Some of mine are: terminal illness, family, brain surgeries, marriage, lumbar punctures, travel, shunts, cats, hemorrhage, faith, and Idiopathic intracranial hypertension. This book is about everything that makes me who I am, and how my life transformed when those three words started this journey.

Some would characterise my journey as unfortunate, but I wouldn't; I'm fortunate to be writing this right now. Instead of dwelling on the darkness, we should be savouring the sun- no matter how fleeting the beam.

Messages for Elise

'For years I had wondered why her? She was just a normal teenage girl. Why right then? She was only 14 and had her whole life ahead of her. What made her so different that she woke up ill on May 25, 2013? I remember begging God to take this pain from her and give it to me. My husband, Steve, did the same. He never gave us what we asked for. Watching her suffer was an extremely painful way to cause me heartache. It was almost as if I stood outside my own body in a fog of doctor appointments, IVs, spinal taps, and rejections. All the while I was watching my precious, young daughter whither away into a diagnosis and no longer a girl with a beautiful name to match her bright blue eyes. I was once reminded by my cousin, Sandra, that the Bible speaks of "angels unawares" and she felt Elise was one.

"Be not forgetful to entertain strangers: for thereby some have entertained angels unawares." - Hebrews 13:2 KJV.

I have felt Elise was truly given this life, not because she was strong enough, but because she was the only one who could. The amount of graciousness, forgiveness, goodness, kindness, and compassion that pours from her heart is unfathomable once you truly realize the amount of pain she suffers. Girls like Elise do not grow up to be just regular women. They grow up to be a warrior princess who wears her battle scars with pride. When people have told her "We will pray God heals you", she has always insisted that they "pray God uses her because maybe healed she's unusable for His glory.'" - **Jackie Fulk (Mom)**

***

'In school, I always heard about how important your attitude is. It wasn't until I lived with Elise that I truly understood what it meant. I've seen her at her highest highs and lowest lows but she's always kept her head held up high. As you may or may not learn in the proceeding book, though a few years apart in age, we weren't close growing up. That only happened with the death of my mother in 2019. While a tragic time that was for me, and most assuredly for everyone else, it spawned a beautiful relationship between me and Elise, and knowing how close it might have never happened is enough to make me weep. Elise, I love you so much and I couldn't be more proud.' – **Jacob Bolling (cousin)**

***

'Elise has made my son Aaron one of the luckiest men in the world. However, can I say this? "Both Aaron and Elise each won the match!" Elise's gift to the world is that she has given both our family and the world the life of a Christian spirit and lovely character. She brings joy to all who know her. The way she manages her health concerns is truly a gift from God. Why then would I say she won the match? Because Aaron has taken on the issue of her health without a moment of regret or a desire for a less complicated life. Yes, she is the winner. Why then, would I say that Aaron won the match? Elise once sent me this meme: "Is it rude to start asking my Mother-in-Law for daily childcare fees? Her child

is a handful and I don't work for free." Aaron, much like me, brings
an abundance of opinion, tenacity, passion, and a lack of filter. I am
delighted he found someone who would accept that, and undeniably love
him. Yes, he is the winner.' - **Gail Goetzinger (Mother-in-law)**

***

It's not very often you come across a situation or person that you
immediately think, someone should write a story about this, but I have
found this in Elise. She has endured unimaginable adversity, yet still
loves the Lord! Elise came to us a couple of years ago wanting a job caring
for our disabled daughter. She told us she was sick and usually had a
surgery or two every year. She would be gone for a few weeks and then
come back to work. After having Elise working for us for a couple of
years, and having several surgeries during that time, I would say that
Elise is a living miracle! Elise has proven her resiliency and has overcome
many struggles during this time, yet her faith in God is still very strong.
I'm glad she has written this book to tell others how God can help them
through difficult times in their life. God has not promised us an easy life,
but what He did promise is that He will be with us as we walk through
this life of difficulties. As we deal with failure, pain, and struggles, we
will grow stronger in our faith and become closer to Him. Elise has shown
me that even though people may seem normal and fine on the outside, on
the inside they can really be struggling or have serious health issues. She
has also shown me that as much as I think my struggles and issues are
difficult, compared to others, mine are nothing to even talk about.

"Joshua 1:9 – Be strong and courageous! Do not be afraid or discour-
aged. For the Lord your God is with you wherever you go."

"Isaiah 41:10 – Fear not, for I am with you; be not dismayed, for I am your God; I will strengthen you, I will help you, I will uphold you with my righteous right hand."' - **Diann Ellington (Boss)**

***

'Let me start by saying this "Someone else always has it harder." I first met Elise in the summer of 2019. I was at the peak of my depression and had just moved to Oregon to get a fresh start and reinvent myself, one might say I was in a "woe is me" era of my life. By the grace of all things good, Elise and I had stumbled across each other. She was happy, sassy, and smart. We slowly started becoming friends and then soon we were inseparable. We shared a lot in common with hardships except for one huge difference, Elise was never upset about what was going on in her life, she never wished it away, she never got angry and she always kept a positive spin on things. Throughout our friendship, she has shown me nothing but positivity and smiles, even while in a hospital bed pending the unknown. I've sat crying my eyes out scared about not knowing what's next and you know what she says to me? Someone else has it worse than she does. Elise has taught me to love and to forgive, how to cope with things, and how to be a better person. If it weren't for her and how she handles things that are thrown at her, I don't think I would've learned what I needed to grow. She's a teacher without knowing it. If you're ever lucky to meet her, you'll see what a strong, amazing, and happy person she is. People come into your life for all sorts of reasons and I firmly believe Elise came into mine and everyone she knows to show that it doesn't matter what's going on in your life, big, small, or somewhere in between, there's* *always room for kindness and to be grateful for what you have.' - **Erika Stewart (Friend)***

***

'Elise walked into my life as a sick, young woman at bible study. I sat next to her for 90 minutes per week. We shared our struggles as two young adults and leaned on our peers, but eventually on each other. Minutes became hours. I began to see an incredible woman. We found each other connecting outside of bible study and soon, I asked her out. Hours became days. I began to admire Elise and wonder how she could have the strength to live and the overflow to share with her friends, family, and me. She inspired me and I started to fall for her. Days became weeks. We walked and we talked and I accompanied her for a few surgeries, and saw her inner soul. Our journey traveled us through good moments, sad moments, and eventually engagement. Weeks became months, months became years. We married outside in June in Western Oregon and there wasn't a raindrop in the sky, and the weather was clear. As I write this, we approach our third wedding anniversary and we have known each other for over 6 years. I haven't ever looked up to a person like Elise. I haven't ever admired anyone like this. And to see the strength God has given her is humbling. I am so blessed and I will forever be in debt to my Lord and Savior for the gifts I have in life, the grandest being Elise.

Now years can become decades and decades will become forever.' - **Aaron Goetzinger (Husband)**

Chapter One

My name is Elise Goetzinger and I have survived 26 brain surgeries.

I have a rare condition called Idiopathic Intracranial Hypertension (IIH) and Chiari. Tomorrow is never promised to any of us, but when you go from being a fun-loving teenager to needing a few brain surgeries per year, you see life differently. My family, my kind-hearted husband and his jokes, my cats, my work, and my travels have helped me to adapt to this new life. I've learned so much and come so far, but now my story needs to be told.

I was born in Houston, Texas, and moved to Colorado for my dad's job in the oil field before relocating again to Wyoming. We lived in Pinedale, a tiny town nestled between snowy mountains, where my parents ran a restaurant called the Patio Grill. When I was eighteen, we settled in Oregon, but I'll always call Wyoming home. After my parent's divorce, I was raised by my mom and stepdad, Steve, with my older sister Olivia, and younger sister Emilie, who was adopted at birth when I was 10 and quickly became my best friend.

My life was pretty ordinary up until I was a freshman in high school. I adored Mathematics and would tutor the upperclassmen in it, but I hated English, science, and the timed miles in P.E. class. Thankfully, my mom agreed that P.E. was pointless, so she would write me notes with the best excuses. I had a group of friends who invigorated our ancient little town. Pinedale didn't even have traffic lights, but it did have a library room with heated floors, computers, and a Wii. So, naturally, we hung out there, posting computer selfies on our Myspace pages. Every summer night, we played cops and robbers with the upperclassmen chasing us through town in their cars, and whenever there were traffic cones laid out, we would reroute them. To top off our mischief, Olivia and I would prank call people so often that one morning the cops turned up at our parents' restaurant to scare us into behaving. Even though we had to travel to Big Piney for a cinema or bowling alley, our town had bonfires, mudding every time the snow melted, and a sense of community that would never leave me.

Around the age of thirteen, I was struggling with awful periods that lasted too long and came too often, so the doctor suggested birth control injections and unfortunately, I said yes. Not long after the first injection, I started to show signs of something being wrong, we just didn't realize it. Almost every time I went to school, I would forget something important like my jacket or lunchbox, and every time, I would have to call my mom and ask her to bring it to me. She used to get so frustrated and launch into a full mom lecture, but how was she to know why I kept forgetting? One time, I had to announce the lineup at a choir concert and the teacher forbade us from taking scripts on stage. I stood in front of the audience and my lines had vanished. I fumbled with the words 'This is the Pinedale...High school choir... uhm', until the teacher stopped screaming at me from off stage and pulled me out of the spotlight. My cheeks burned with embarrassment, and I couldn't explain that I had learned my lines, because if I had, where were they?

The first time something really seemed to be wrong was on a very important day. My mom and stepdad had just gotten married at their wedding in January 2012, and my head started throbbing until my vision disappeared and I dropped to the ground. I don't remember what happened after that, it's like my memory of that beautiful day faded to black. I thought it was a one-time thing, just a horrible little blip, but then it happened again. We were on the computers at school, assessing our rank in the class, and I was looking at my computer when all of a sudden, it disappeared and I couldn't see my friends, the teacher, or the room. The teacher phoned my mom, and my stepdad came to carry me out of the school, with the help of the principal. Again, my memory drifted away, leaving me with another blank space in my childhood. I knew something was wrong at that point, but what? Normality resumed again, but not for long.

I had just made a 4.0 GPA with a few other classmates, and we were rewarded with a visit to an amazing theme park before singing in the choir for the graduating class that night. The whole day is clouded over, but I have a small, dim picture of standing in the choir amongst kids in green caps and gowns. The next day was Saturday, May 25th, 2013, and I have no recollection of it, but apparently, at 9 am, I threw my mom's bedroom door open and stumbled in, startling her awake. With huge black pupils consuming all the blue in my eyes, I said I was numb from top to bottom on my right side, had a terrible headache, and felt nauseous. My mom was terrified and called her friend Windi, a life-flight nurse, who told my mom to rush me to the hospital as fast as possible. So, she dropped everything and took me to the Pinedale Medical Clinic. Everybody assumed it was drugs at first, but I was only fourteen years old. The clinic gave me a 'migraine cocktail', but no answers. A kind, sweet little old lady treated me, and that took some of my fear away. But two more ineffective migraine cocktails later, we went to St. John's Health in Jackson. At first, they didn't know what to do with me, so they tried some uncommon medications like

D.H.E. 45, but none of them helped. By Monday, May 27th, I was in a comatose state and had to be life-flighted to Salt Lake City Primary Children's Hospital. At 11 am, my stepdad and sisters visited before we left, and there's a photograph of us in which my eyes look empty. At that point, I didn't know my colors, numbers, or anything, and what was more concerning was that I could barely recognize people.

Mom and I stayed at the Children's Hospital for over two weeks… not exactly the holiday either of us had in mind. Their first assumptions were that I had a bleed on the brain, or that someone from school or the amusement park had drugged me, even though the effects would have worn off by then. While they called poison control for advice, my mom searched me for a tick bite bullseye rash in case I had Lyme disease. The doctor also said that I had 'halos' around my pupils but no papilledema- not that we understood what that meant. They got speech therapists to assess me, and my family would try playing games, like Uno, but I just stared at the cards blankly. I didn't even know who my dad was, I thought he was a nurse. When all other options had been exhausted, they tried a bedside blind Lumbar Puncture (spinal tap). This measures the cerebrospinal fluid (CSF) pressure, and my opening pressure was 22 (that's considered high and is key in diagnosing IIH), but because the fluid was clear, they said nothing was wrong with me. My mom was told by the doctor that 22 was not high-pressure and only 30 upwards was considered high, and she couldn't argue with that.

Not long after, I woke up to find myself in a pitch-black room. The only light came from the phone that illuminated my mom's crying face, but as soon as she heard my voice asking where we were, her face truly lit up. That face was the best one that I could have woken up to, but it was shattering to hear what was happening to me. I had been catheterized since the life flight because I had no idea how to use the toilet, but after the spinal tap, I asked for it to be taken out because I felt better, and my head didn't hurt as much. As soon as a young nurse heard that the spinal tap had made me feel better, she knew something wasn't right. She whispered to my mom that they were wrong because opening pressure should never be above 15, and I'm grateful that she spoke up and told my mom to research it.

We were quickly sent home with no help, and although I was responsive, I was still sick. I started throwing up constantly and my mom knew that something had to be done. She found a naturopathic specialist who was based in Big Piney at the time. We went to see this new doctor who investigated every inch of my body before sending us away while she made some phone calls. Later that day, she told us to quickly pack some bags because she was arranging a life flight to Denver Children's Hospital.

When we got to Denver, my mom and I waited in a large hospital room until a female neurologist and two student doctors came in; one tall man and one young woman.

This neurologist checked me over from head to toe and then turned to my mom and said 'There is nothing wrong with your daughter. She is just…' and she spun her finger around to say crazy.

My mom later told me that her instinctive reaction was rage; she couldn't believe that anybody would say such an unimaginably vile thing in front of me. Before her fury bubbled over, she turned to me and saw huge doe eyes, brimming with tears, staring at her helplessly, and she knew that at that moment, I just needed my mom.

We were asked to leave, so my mom bit her tongue and simply said, 'We are not leaving this room until my husband gets here and that's a six-hour drive'.

While we were waiting for my stepdad, Mom was weeping on the phone to my aunt, and I was getting one final check-up by the head nurse. By some miracle, I suddenly had a high fever so they had to admit me.

The next morning, a lovely hospitalist, Barry, brought some students into my room and told them that my CAT scan had shown inflamed sinuses. Thank God for that sinus infection. We told that sweet man my entire story and he said that if the headache persisted after the sinus infection, I would need another spinal tap. He agreed that it sounded like IIH was the underlying issue. In the following years, seeing Barry became the only enjoyable part of visiting Denver Children's Hospital.

Not long after we returned home, I became unwell again. The naturopathic specialist told us to go to Big Piney ER. Mom drove me there straight away, as I was very pale, confused, and had low blood pressure. We were quickly told that I had sepsis, but it was just a small ER, so I had to take an ambulance to Salt Lake City Hospital. Mom asked if she could meet Steve to collect some essentials, and then get into the ambulance where it would pass by on its way to Salt Lake City, and they said yes. So, my mom set off, and they started the ambulance journey while stabilizing me with fluids. Everything was going to plan until I started crashing, fast. My whole body turned ice-cold, and I was no longer lucid. My blood pressure began dropping dangerously low, and it wouldn't come back up no matter what they tried, so the paramedics called for a life flight. When my mom heard the news, she slammed her foot down, put her hazard lights on, and called 911 to inform them of her reasoning in case they pulled her over. She later said that if a cop did attempt to pull her over, she would have kept driving until she reached me and then dealt with the consequences later. Thankfully, she arrived just in time for the life flight to take us to the hospital. I was pumped with countless bags of fluids and antibiotics, and after a two-week stay, I was finally able to go home. Of course, when we got home, the original headaches persisted. As Barry suggested, I visited our trusted primary care physician to get another spinal tap and this time, it showed a pressure of 35. I finally got the diagnosis of IIH that we had been looking for. Due to my extra issues, I was also tested for Ehlers-Danlos syndrome, but I was two little points off diagnosis. However, an IIH diagnosis is what we had been praying for. It wasn't an ideal situation, but IIH needs to be acknowledged and treated correctly otherwise it can be fatal.

Diagnosis day was a pivotal point in my life. After that, the hospital appointments began to pile up until I had no option but to quit the school that I barely got to see anymore. Although, with rumors flying around about me faking my illness, school was just a breeding ground for bullies. Even though I had a 504 plan that should have protected me from anything to do with disability, the school threatened to take my mom to court unless my attendance improved. Nothing made me well enough to go to school, so my mom had no choice but to homeschool. We got a tutor, but I was drowning in schoolwork, and it was impossible to catch up on everything. Despite our best efforts, my hopes of returning to normality began to crumble in front of me. The only thing that kept my days bright was the daycare I worked at. After dropping out of school, I needed something to do on the days I was well enough to do anything. Most of my friends were twice my age because the rumors at school meant that teenagers bullied me-some until restraining orders were needed. My older friend's mom ran a daycare center and she let me work with the 2-4-year-olds. The happiness radiating from those kids made everything feel okay and I adored every day that I worked there until we moved to Oregon.

For a while after the initial diagnosis, I was bounced back and forth between Salt Lake and Denver Children's Hospital. Salt Lake refused to believe the diagnosis and Denver wasn't willing to help me unless it was so bad that I was going blind. So, it was still a battle to get the help that I needed. The rest of my childhood was enveloped in hospital rooms and the majority of my friends deserted or bullied me. Instead of a first kiss, first prom, or first homecoming, I had a first spinal tap, first life flight, and first hearing aid. While other girls curled their hair for prom, I shaved mine for brain surgery. The memories of my previous life faded until barely anything remained. Yet for every appointment, my mom wrapped her hands in mine and got me through it until I adapted to this new notion of life.

Chapter Two

In October 2013, a doctor told my mom that I would be better within a year, but by that point, I had already been in a 48-hour induced coma and tried treatments like acupuncture and Botox. However, Botox caused pressure in the back of my skull and migraines, and a while later a doctor in Idaho Falls explained that Botox is one of the worst things you can do for IIH. Since May, my mom had been asking the Primary Children's Hospital for an MRV (magnetic resonance venography) to search for a cause of the IIH. In December, we stayed in Salt Lake City for a few days while they did an MRV, MRI, and neurocognitive testing. They didn't provide any answers.

My first brain surgery was the placement of an Intracranial Pressure Monitoring bolt in March 2014. I had already tried Diamox and similar medications that reduce brain pressure but found that I'm allergic to them and they turned my skin yellow, meaning medication wasn't an option for me. So, we went to see a specialist named Dr. Rahman in Portland, Oregon. A very kind family let us stay with them for over a month in their floating home- a concept that I found fascinating until I moved to Oregon and found that they're quite unexceptional things. At OHSU, Dr. Rahman began by checking my vision. However, the first thing to go has always been my hearing. I lost 75% of the hearing in my right ear during the first life flight, so I often get my hearing checked now. Next, they did an MRA (Magnetic resonance angiography), which came back fine. They also did a cerebral angiogram. That was to check the structure of the blood vessels in my brain to ensure there were no issues like clots. Normally they put you to sleep or dose you up with sedatives, but I just asked for light numbing. It was difficult to perform the procedure because I was tiny, and they struggled to get the agent from my groin all the way up to my neck. They constantly checked if I was alright, but honestly, I was fine because that pain was nothing compared to what I had been going through. When telling my mom that they hadn't found anything, they also mentioned that anybody would have passed out with that level of pain, and they couldn't figure out why I didn't. My stepdad recently underwent the same procedure and even though he wanted to stay awake as I had done, he had to be sedated. He called me afterward saying that he had no idea how I had done it.

Finally, Dr. Rahman decided to confirm my diagnosis with an ICP bolt. This is a procedure where they drill into the skull and insert a catheter to measure CSF pressure for 48-72 hours. I had to be conscious so that they would know if something was going wrong. My mom sat opposite me, her face trembling as she wiped the blood away before it could drip down my face. I'll never forget the sound of that drill penetrating my skull. Once the bolt was in place, they noticed that when I was lying down it was 25-40, but when I stood up it spiked to 60-100, which made Dr. Rahman so nervous that he told me to stay lying down. After 48 hours, they removed it and then came the discussion of what would happen next. My mom suggested a shunt (an internal device that drains the excess CSF), but the doctor refused because I was so young and small. Of course, a shunt doesn't grow with you so it's not the best option for a growing fifteen-year-old.

My mom asked, 'What is she supposed to do then, lay down forever?'

The only solution that he could think of was to keep doing spinal taps to relieve the pressure until I was older. So, from March to October, I had countless. I was having three spinal taps per week plus injections to help with the pain.

In June 2014, my mom found a neurologist in Idaho Falls who was willing to take me on. We walked into his office assuming it would be a quick visit never to be repeated, like all of the other failed attempts. However, he spent over 2 hours talking *to* me- not about me or for me.

He asked, 'What is wrong with you?'

I replied, 'I have IIH?'

He asked, 'Do you know why the back of your head hurts?', and I said no.

He replied, 'Because you have IIH'.

My mom and I burst into tears because someone who could help me had believed me. The doctor offered to give me trigger point injections for the pain, but it wasn't long after that I needed another spinal tap.

After months of these health issues, my stepdad Steve decided to cheer me up with our favorite hobby. I had always been good at rifle hunting and bow shooting. Before I got sick I wanted to be a sniper in the Marines because long-range rifle hunting was where my talent shone, but with my health, they could never accept me. Steve was my hunting buddy and we used to go almost every weekend so when we saw that there was a bow shooting contest, it was a welcome distraction. I joined the female contest and Steve joined the male one. Neither of us expected to win anything and it was just for fun, which is why I was very surprised when I got first place. I thought maybe I'd win $50 but I won an expensive week-long hunting trip with guide

Mike Schmid, a well-known hunter with a YouTube channel called 'Intrepid Outdoors' and a TV show. I asked if I could bring someone with me but I was underage so I had to and I immediately picked Steve. Excitement kept my mind occupied during every hospital appointment until our trip in September.

A couple of weeks before the trip, rain hammered down on the car as my mom and stepdad drove me to Idaho Falls. My symptoms had gotten worse again and I couldn't stop vomiting with excruciating pressure pain. The doctor gave me Phenergan and Toradol then sent me across the street to the main hospital for a spinal tap. That one had an opening pressure of 50, which made the doctor take me even more seriously because he had never seen such a high pressure. He said that if I needed any more spinal taps, he would arrange them so that we didn't have to travel all that way, which was beyond helpful. What was even more helpful was that he found gold dust- a neurosurgeon willing to perform my shunt surgery.

The pressure symptoms calmed down enough for Steve and me to drive to Devil's Tower for the hunting trip. On September 10th, we arrived at a ginormous ranch in the beautiful wilderness of Wyoming. There was so much to explore and they had activities like ATV driving which kept Steve entertained while I hunted. Not only was I the youngest there but I was the only female, which felt weird. There was one kid who was only a little older than me so we became fast friends. We quickly made it into a competition for who could catch the biggest buck. The guide, Mike, said that I could choose between a buck, or a mountain lion and I had never seen a real mountain lion so obviously I wanted to catch one. They were the hardest to catch, so he made the compromise that if I got a buck and had time to spare, I could try to get one of each. He explained that the camera crew might be extra interested in getting my perspective because I was the only girl.

I was just shocked when he said camera crew because I had no idea I would end up on a TV show too. Steve couldn't come hunting with me because Mike and I picked a tree blind that barely had room for the two of us, but the ATVs kept him happy. Mike and I hiked to the tree blind at 4 am for four mornings in a row. It was exhausting but words couldn't describe how lucky I felt. On day one Mike spotted a pretty big buck, but I wanted bigger. We came back on day two to find the same buck, but I still wanted to wait for the perfect one. On day three, I was using my tiny binoculars to watch the buck in the forest and noticed that Mike had fallen asleep next to me. I let him sleep until lunch and he was mortified that he'd fallen asleep. We went back in the evening and that same big buck was there taunting me because I still hadn't seen a bigger one. On the fourth day, the same buck returned, but with it came a bigger one. Mike told me to pick one of the big ones and I picked the biggest. After I shot him, I started crying, and when Mike asked me why, I said I was so proud of how well I had done. After all I had been through recently, I was just proud of myself for getting through the trip and accomplishing my goal.

Mike asked what I wanted to do next, assuming I would want to go to sleep but I replied, 'Duh, we're gonna go eat it!'

We called Mike's people, along with Steve, to come and get us and the buck. We were about 6 miles into the woods, so a truck was needed to transport this huge buck back to camp.

When Steve saw it, he said 'It's so big! You even got it in the perfect spot!'

I adored making him proud. That arrow remained perfectly intact, so it now lies on top of the buck's antlers. When the other kid and I compared our bucks, his was maybe a fraction of an inch larger, so he insisted he won but I definitely won with that shot. After that, Mike asked if I wanted to use my last two days to get a mountain lion, but I just wanted to relax and take in the ranch with Steve instead. It was an amazing experience and just what I needed at that moment in time.

Chapter Three

On Halloween 2014, it finally happened. A neurosurgeon in Idaho agreed to do VP (ventriculoperitoneal) shunt surgery and even though it was a long journey, my entire family came to be with me for the little time that they could. Then it was just my mom and me again, and even though I missed my little sister every second of each day, I was starting to get used to it being just the two of us. A friend of my mom's, Janice, made me a quilt of pink patches, each with their own bright designs of polka dots, sprinkled cupcakes, and swirly lollipops. It came to countless hospitals as my comforting good luck charm, and I still cherish it, but now my husband is the charm that comes with me instead.

Before the surgery, my mom took me to the hairdressers at a mall and had to ask if they would shave my head. The hospital said that hair increases the risk of infection, but I know now that they only need to shave the incision area, so I protect the rest by braiding it. A lovely woman welcomed me into the salon, and we shared a beautiful moment as she shaved my hair and we cried together. Words can't describe how it felt to be a sixteen-year-old girl having to sacrifice a part of my identity and that innate idea of beauty.

The surgery got off to a rocky start, as they covered me in chlorhexidine, without realizing that I was allergic to it. My skin burned red, and I puffed up like the girl from *Willy Wonka*. It took four Epi-pens to stop the allergic reaction. This one is a tricky allergy for someone who has surgery often, as the surgeons even wash their hands with it and if they nick their gloves, I'll react to it. Eventually, the surgery went ahead, but the recovery was equally as terrible as the start; I even got cauliflower ear. Nonetheless, I was so grateful to the surgeon who allowed the shunt.

At the beginning of 2015, I found myself searching for something fun. A friend had recently entered Miss Teen Wyoming and it sounded amazing, so I googled 'beauty pageants near me' and found Our Little Miss. I entered the trial pageant and won, although my main competition clearly didn't want to be there, so I didn't have to try too hard to win. I'd tried something new, and it was fun, but I was satisfied. What I didn't know was that if you win the trial, you have to do the universal pageant and go up against people from different states and countries, even as far as China. There was one girl from my age category that I immediately knew would win. She was kind and gorgeous, like a Barbie doll without a single strand of hair out of line. I felt inferior and like I'd be one of the first to go... I barely had any hair after all. The pageant director got mad at me for spiking my tufts of hair up into a little mohawk, but what else could I do with it? None of it mattered anyway, I knew that girl would win, and she deserved it. This was just a bit of fun, a distraction from the mundane days of illness.

I always preferred the kind, unjudging company of little kids to teenagers my age, so while everyone was socializing I hung out with the kids. The judges were always assessing us, and they noticed that I was the only one who chose to go and have fun with the little ones instead of standing around awkwardly like the other teens. Eventually, I was told to line up on stage in front of the judges with five other girls. I was third in line.

They asked the first girl 'What do you like to do for fun?'

She said 'Shopping.'

The next girl was asked 'If you had a million dollars, what would you do?'

She replied, 'I'd go straight to the mall.'

They repeated 'If you had a million dollars, what would you do?'

I said, 'I'd give it to my dad so he could pay my medical bills.'

They looked puzzled and asked what I meant. I explained that my hair wasn't shaved by choice and that I'd had two brain surgeries, life flights, and a bunch of other costly things. When it was time to find out who won, they narrowed it down to the top ten and I was still there. So, I thought *I'll be tenth, that's great*. When they reached fifth I thought *Okay, I must be fifth, that's amazing*. When they reached second, I realized the only other girl was the one who would win.

I smiled at her and said 'I'm so glad that you won!'

As I said that, they called her name, and she received her second-place award. I dropped to the ground with tears of shock and gratitude. I couldn't believe that something so wonderful would happen to me and I couldn't understand why. The gorgeous girl who came second hugged me with a genuine smile and demonstrated how women should support each other which made that moment even more special. There had been three judges and the old man who sat in the middle introduced himself to me afterwards. Mel explained that he had seen how different I was when I played with the children and after he heard about my illness, he said to the other judges that he would give up his vote for every other category as long as I got first place in mine. I stayed in touch with Mel until his recent death. He would call me his granddaughter and meet me at the few pageant events that I managed to attend afterwards. He was the most delightful man, and I was beyond grateful for his kindness on that momentous winter day.

A couple of months later, something felt wrong. After a while of returning symptoms, I saw the surgeon, Dr. Coin. He did an X-ray and found no kinks or clogs in the shunt, so he blamed all of the headaches, hearing loss, blurry vision, and nausea on migraines. A few weeks later, my mom called him again. They did another X-ray that showed nothing and a visual field that showed massive deterioration of my vision. We asked for an MRI because I just knew something was wrong with the shunt, but that looked fine too. They did a shunt tap which proved I had raised pressure and convinced him to take me seriously. A nuclear medicine study showed that the valve in my shunt was broken, and it gave us the extra surprise of an enlarged appendix.

Dr. Coin simply said, 'Shunts don't break'.

But it had. On May 2nd, 2015, he 'fixed' the shunt via surgery, removed my appendix, and then refused to perform surgery on me again. His hands were trembling as he 'tapped' the shunt, which makes sense considering shunt taps can puncture the valve and break it even more. That's exactly what happened. We didn't realize it at the time, but he probably had no idea what he was doing. I had assumed that Dr. Coin was going to be my neurosurgeon forever. Instead of feeling dejected like my mom, I told myself I wouldn't need him again anyway because if shunts don't break then it must have been a one-off.

Chapter Four

Halfway into 2015, my mom began tirelessly searching for a new neurosurgeon who was willing to take me on. She joined an IIH support group, and a bunch of people suggested Dr. Knives, a surgeon in Las Vegas, Nevada. Even though this was very far away from us, we were desperate, so my mom called, emailed, and sent letters to his office until they agreed to see me. I had just turned seventeen, and on my little sister's birthday on July 22nd, 2015, I got my second VP shunt revision. I felt awful that my mom and I were in Nevada on Emilie's birthday, but we had no choice and Dr. Knives was the most promising neurosurgeon. He used to ask me what I wanted when I got out of surgery and one time I really craved Showboy Bake Shop cupcakes, so he went to collect about two dozen of them. Whatever treat I requested was always sitting on a tray waiting for me after surgery. Traveling to Nevada each time I needed a revision was awful but thankfully, the Ronald McDonald house let my mom and I stay there. That charity was wonderful. We stayed there for months at a time, because I had surgery in July, two in September, and another in October so we couldn't leave.

During those months, I spent most of my time either in the hospital or at the Ronald McDonald house. The accommodation gave us breakfast and dinner, but when we had to stay in the hospital, the food was disgusting. My mom would go and get us takeout sometimes, but she didn't want to leave me alone most of the time. Once, the nurses showed up with two big boxes of pizza for us, which was incredibly kind. Mom would also bring her own sheets, pillows, and egg crate mattress topper so that she could sleep on the hospital couch if I'd just had surgery. She was very prepared by that point.

Las Vegas wasn't exactly the perfect place for a bored, sick teenager and the mom in charge who didn't drink, but we found our own fun. We got to explore quite a lot within a couple of weeks before the first surgery. We had to stay there for that time because we went back and forth to the hospital for the preparatory scans and tests. Mom and I went to get Sonic most nights because I always have and always will crave their tator tots with cheese and a vanilla Coke. Late one night, we drove past a college on the way to get food and ten tiny bunnies ran in front of the car. Our eyes followed them as they blended into an enormous crowd of bunnies in the field across from the college. There must have been a thousand of them.

Mom and I looked at each other and she said, 'Did you see that?'

'The bunnies? Yeah.'

'Oh, so I'm not crazy,' she laughed.

We continued driving, both wondering why there was a huge horde of bunnies in the middle of Las Vegas. On the way back to the Ronald McDonald house, we passed by the college again and the cute crowd was still there. We got out of the car and let their fluffy goodness swarm us. Las Vegas didn't provide tons of nature for them to feed off, so Mom suggested that we buy them some nutritious food. After petting them for a while, we headed to Target and brought back a load of vegetables. This became our nightly tradition, and I adored it. When I couldn't leave the hospital, my mom would do it alone and film them for me. When Emilie and my stepdad were able to visit, Emilie would get so excited about seeing 'Elise's bunnies'. Someone at the Ronald McDonald house overheard us talking about the bunnies and told us that they were the college's experimentation animals. Nothing harmful apparently, but once the students had done their tests, they released the bunnies into the field. So, the bizarre bunny horde was explained.

Another vivid memory is when I was so lethargic that I could barely walk, but I wanted to get out of the same four hospital walls for a while. So, my mom put me in a wheelchair and took me to a wildlife park. Everyone was getting in the water to swim with the dolphins, but I couldn't. A lovely employee helped me out of the wheelchair so that I could pet and feed them instead. She also gave us a private tour around the rest of the park, and we got to see animals up close that only employees could- that was an amazing act of inclusion.

Around October time, we visited a bunch of haunted houses and found one that claimed to be the scariest. Of course, we didn't believe that, but when an exceptionally creepy man jumped out at us, I pushed my mom towards him and ran away. She sat dazed on the floor watching my screaming figure fade into the distance and the creepy man helped her up. For some reason, everyone refuses to go into haunted houses with me now.

One of the VP shunt revisions in September 2015 was needed because the shunt catheter had broken. I have unusually narrow ventricles in my brain, and I still have a few broken catheters in there now because they got stuck, and pulling them out would risk causing a stroke (we'll get to that later). I am now down to one of the last ventricles for a catheter to go into, so I'm praying that this one never breaks. September 22nd, 2015 was the third annual IIH awareness day since I had been diagnosed in June 2013 and it was ironically my third year of having it. By that point, I'd had countless spinal taps, forty hospital stays, four life flights, and the list goes on. However, it finally felt like we were getting somewhere with the medical support I was receiving. Dr. Knives was one of the best neurosurgeons I've ever met, and he was the one who recommended me for Make-A-Wish. This was because I'm terminally ill and they never thought I would make it past twenty-five. When I first wrote this, I was twenty-five and thankful to be proving them wrong. As I publish this, I'm twenty-six and incredibly grateful that I'm still proving them wrong.) I had a representative in Wyoming who helped me make my wish to go to Ukraine. However, I kept having surgeries and the trip kept getting postponed. When I moved to Oregon, I got a brilliant new representative named Jessica, but my wish had to be altered again because I wasn't allowed to fly at that point.

Visiting Ukraine was my first wish because I had roots there. My Babusia (great-grandmother), Dadusia (great-grandfather), and Nana lived there during the Second World War. When my Nana was young, she had to stay in a German hospital, and she learned to speak the language well. After she was discharged, she and Babusia were about to board the train home and were stopped by a German soldier who was asking where they were going.

Babusia would have sensibly lied in German about where they were going, but he turned to my Nana and said, 'I was asking her.'

Thankfully, she replied in German. Unfortunately, they later ended up in a concentration camp and I remember the stories my Nana used to tell me, like how they hid under creaking tables as bombs hit. I was incredibly close with my Nana, and I adored flying to Texas to visit her. She would say I was her heartbeat and sing 'You are my sunshine' to me. It was a once-in-a-lifetime bond. Not long after I got sick, she died. My friend threw me a fake prom because I had missed the real one and my Nana was staying with us, but she insisted that I go and have some fun. I left for one night and the next morning, I found that she had passed away on my bedroom floor from a stress-induced heart attack. I was devastated beyond words and couldn't stay in my house for weeks afterward. Although, I was grateful that she didn't have to go through the heartbreak of watching me suffer through all of those surgeries. Side note- my mom allowed me to get a tattoo in her memory and for my first tattoo, I picked the rib cage- never pick the rib cage.

So, I made that wish because I wanted to see where my Nana's stories came from, step on the soil that she grew up on, and feel close to her again. In February 2018, three years after the original idea, Make-A-Wish granted the alternative wish of going on a beautiful cruise. I was nineteen but I still had to wear a badge that said, 'I'm a Make-A-Wish kid', so I stuck 'adult' over the last word and made the badge my own.

While those months in Las Vegas were primarily hospital beds and surgeries, there were many beautiful highlights. Due to those months, Ronald McDonald and Make-A-Wish are two charities I will always donate to and forever be grateful for. That gratitude extends to Dr. Knives and although I hoped he would always be my surgeon, the next year was my last surgery with him.

Chapter Five

A fter months in Las Vegas, I was home in time for 2015 to end with a bang. On the 22nd of November, my parents were at St. John's Health in Jackson for the day because my stepdad had just had surgery on his shoulder. I was looking after Emilie, but I was called to go to Big Piney to collect jaw images in preparation for having my wisdom teeth out. A blizzard was raging outside so I thought it safest to drop Emilie off with our family friends the Danielses. I dropped her off, drove to Big Piney, and on the way back, I could barely see two feet in front of me- everything was white. I called my mom from the car while hunched over the steering wheel like an old lady, driving about 10mph. I told them to not drive home until the blizzard died down and my mom agreed. Suddenly I hit a patch of black ice, lost control of the tires, and had to choose between crashing into the oncoming traffic or going off the road. I tried to steer away from the traffic, but I fishtailed and ended up about 550ft off the road, down a steep drop, and crashing into a huge deer fence pole. It came through the back window and out of the front- directly through where Emilie would have been sitting. I can't even think about what would have happened if she weren't at the Daniel's. My mom was still on the phone, but I couldn't hear her. I was worried that nobody had seen it, so I busted open my window and crawled out of the car and up the hill until I reached the road. The snow burnt my skin as I dug my way up the hill in just a t-shirt, jeans, and boots. Once I saw headlights and felt the road, I collapsed and waited for help. Some very kind truck drivers wrapped me up in blankets, called 911, and told me to not move.

My head was swimming, but I managed to say, 'I just had brain surgery a few months ago. Call my mom'.

When the ambulance and police turned up, one of the policemen recognized me and he knew my family and my situation, so he insisted on staying with me until we got to St. John's Health. I ended up meeting my mom and stepdad at the hospital with my two broken ribs, bruised tailbone, and concussion.

My stepdad was there in his sling and joked, 'Are you just trying to one-up me?'

Poor Emilie was worried sick. She has always had a high IQ, and even at that young age, she figured out exactly when I should have been back for her and knew something was wrong. Thankfully our friends took good care of her for us that night.

Despite being in considerable pain from the accident, I was invited to take part in something special on December 13th. I got to represent Our Little Miss at the Pinedale Christmas Parade. I wore the tall crown and white sash while bundled up in a glittering sleigh float with the lovely little girl who was Wyoming's Mini Queen. It was wonderful to be a part of that cheerful celebration.

After recovering from the car accident, on January 29th, 2016, I ended up going to Las Vegas for another surgery. On the screens, it said, 'Right frontal ventricular peritoneal shunt revision, insert right frontal camino intracranial pressure monitor via twist drill neuroen-doscope assisted'. Basically, it was a VP shunt revision with an ICP bolt during the procedure to monitor the pressure. We went to Nevada about one week before the surgery, as we always had to, for tests to determine the problem. We stayed in the Ronald McDonald house again and by that point, everyone who worked there knew us pretty well. For this one, almost everybody came with me- my mom, stepdad, and Emilie. Emilie was still so little, and I loved being able to hold her hand while I waited for them to take me into operating room. I was admitted to the hospital a few days before surgery, and we requested one particular night nurse because he was so wonderfully compassionate and would set alarms on his phone so that my painkillers were never a minute late. Dr. Knives believed that a shaved head reduced the risk of infection, but I had just grown a decent length of hair and dyed it blonde, so I wasn't ecstatic about having that little bald head again. During the surgery, they fixed the broken valve and replaced the tubing. Dr. Knives used a new type of small valve imported from France, which was less noticeable beneath my skin. The day after, I was in the PICU, exhausted and struggling with little to no sleep due to unbearable pain. I called Showboy Bake Shop to ask for a cupcake delivery to distract me, but they were one step ahead of me and already had my room number ready to deliver my favorites. I adored those kind boys and their fabulous cupcakes. At the time, this was the most agonizing surgery, and the recovery took much longer than I'd hoped. That thought amuses me now because I didn't know that the more the same area gets cut into, the more painful recovery becomes each time. For example, my recent 25th brain surgery was incredibly difficult to recover from.

Another memory from that surgery is the delightful nun who wandered around the hospital and prayed for anybody who needed it. We weren't of the same religion, but she came to my bedside, held my hand, and wanted to hear anything I had to say. She was such a thoughtful woman, and I deeply appreciated her company.

We had recently discovered that I was allergic to sutures, so I had staples. My mom was given a staple puller by Dr. Knives and he taught her how to remove my staples after the two-week mark so that we could go home before then. We could be pretty convincing doctors with the amount of medical knowledge we've gained by now. Dr. Knives moved away a few months later and regardless of hair shaving, he was a truly wonderful surgeon and human.

By June, I was almost eighteen years old, and my stepdad got a job in Oregon. So, Olivia stayed at college in Wyoming, while my parents, Emilie, and I moved to Oregon. Not long after we had settled in, Olivia came to visit for a few weeks, and I loved feeling like a typical teenager with her for a while. I would drive her around and she would roll the windows down, blast music and scream along while I shrunk into my shell hoping nobody would recognize me afterward. My hair had grown since the last time it was shaved off and Olivia wanted to 'surprise me' by dying it. She picked maroon and as much as I loved it, it definitely wasn't my color.

On October 15th, 2016, I had another VP shunt revision with a new surgeon in Oregon, Dr. Cokinos. Earlier that month, I had been in the bathroom and suddenly I couldn't see. I called my mom in, and she instantly realized why- my eyes were filled with blood. We immediately went to the eye doctor. I was so sick and lethargic that I couldn't even sit in the chair for the first guy to examine me, so they called in the specialist who held my head back, took one look into my eyes, and said I needed to go to the hospital. After calling ahead for us, he noticed that my mom was crying.

He compassionately placed a hand on her knee and asked, 'Are you doing this alone? Do you need help?'

Of course, my stepdad was just at work, but she probably did need help coping with it all by that point.

We went to Riverbend Hospital and found out that toxic substances had built up in my blood and traveled to my brain, causing a serious infection and hepatic encephalopathy. That's when I met my new neurosurgeon, who started me on crazy amounts of antibiotics and wanted to replace my broken shunt before it could get infected completely. Right before I went into surgery, my blood pressure started to drop, so they gave me steroids and the anaesthesiologist reassured my mom that they would be extra vigilant. Then they shaved my head again, so the maroon was no more, and proceeded with the surgery. It sounded like the surgery went to plan, but a couple of days later the symptoms were still there, so they did some imaging. My mom had also started to wonder why Dr. Cokinos hadn't given me a post-op assessment yet. Finally, he turned up with the results of the imaging. He explained that the catheter was not right, and more emergency surgery was needed, but his words sounded rehearsed. Mom realized that his extra careful wording could have been because he had done it wrong and needed to fix his mistake. Again, the surgery sounded like it went fine, and he did not show up for a post-op check. Eventually, a nurse entered, and Dr. Cokinos stood outside the window like a guilty puppy. The nurse said that he wouldn't be treating me anymore and we knew it was to avoid getting into trouble for a mistake. Documents from the surgeries later proved that theory. Since then, people have asked why I never sue the terrible doctors, but it's difficult enough to find someone willing to operate on me, and I don't want to deter them even more.

At the beginning of November, a kind lady called Janna from Mirage Hair Systems alongside the Angel Hair Foundation gave me a wonderful gift. After nine brain surgeries, my hair hadn't been able to grow very much ever since it was first shaved. So, when I was given the gift of long hair (worth around $1000!), I felt like myself again. That was wonderful.

It had been a busy year, and amidst the craziness, everybody failed to mention that the water in Oregon was a lot colder than it looked. One autumn day, I took Emilie to the beach for a peaceful swim and as soon as our toes touched the water, we retreated, shivering in our bathing suits. Christmas that year brought some much-needed cheer. My family has a tradition of picking names out of a hat and then just buying gifts for that one person. However much to my annoyance, everyone still buys me an extra gift. I also got to visit Wyoming at the end of 2016 and rekindle friendships with the couple of good friends that I still had there. Even though the past couple of years had been the most unexpectedly difficult, I was realizing that life was still full of blessings.

Chapter Six

2017 was an important year for me. Not only did I meet my future husband, but I had just one surgery- one I've resented ever since.

I met Aaron at church in the Spring of 2017. He was a few years older than me, but a bunch of the young adults did bible study together, so we knew each other through that. I hated talking about my illness because I just wanted to fit in and feel like everybody else. When I eventually admitted I was unwell during bible study, Aaron could be quite dismissive of it because he didn't understand. It turned out that Aaron had heard all about my illnesses from my stepdad who he sometimes worked with, except he didn't realize it was me.

One time at church, I told Aaron that Steve would be dropping off some stuff at his house and he replied, 'Well why doesn't Steve tell me that himself, how does he even know you?'

It turns out that he deeply respected Steve's daughter after hearing about her struggles and once he realized who that was, he transferred that respect to me. However, after we discussed an appointment that I had around August time it was clear that he didn't fully my illness understand yet.

We found a new neurosurgeon called Dr. McGill in Corvallis. During the summer, I was getting such bad pressure issues, but I wasn't sure why because my shunt didn't feel broken this time. A spinal tap showed a pressure of 30 but the tests proved that my shunt was fine. Dr. McGill adjusted the shunt to the highest drainage, but my pressure remained high. He explained that after a while of having a shunt, the body gets used to it and can create more fluid, which was happening to me. Dr. McGill said that they couldn't use the last brain ventricle, so an LP shunt was the only option. I knew that LP shunts could cause Chiari, so I wanted a VA shunt, but he said no due to my heart issues.

When I spoke to the bible study group about it, Aaron said that an LP shunt would be fine because he had a friend with one and they had no issues. I argued that his friend had one because of hydrocephalus so the circumstances were completely different, and my LP shunt would be more likely to break or cause Chiari.

His response was 'You just got to be more positive'.

I replied, 'I'm a realist', and I would have liked to respond a little differently, but he soon understood.

With no other option, the LP shunt surgery was booked for the end of October, but there was something wonderful booked for before then. I had always called myself the 'Loner child' after my Nana passed away because Olivia was close with my dad, Emilie with my mom, and I had my Nana. However, after the past few years of constant hospital visits with my mom, we grew very close. So, I bought us a 7-day cruise for the 22nd of September, which was the perfect bonding trip and a distraction from the upcoming surgery. We went to Canada, San Francisco, and Astoria, Oregon. Although Alcatraz was by far our favorite excursion.

There was an ex-inmate selling books outside Alcatraz and I took a photo of him and my mom in which he is just staring down her shirt.

I said, 'Can you look at me this time?' before snapping another one.

It was fascinating to see inside the infamous prison and then talk to someone who stayed there. We met a bunch of people on that cruise, including a man called Scott who lives from cruise to cruise- what a life! We took part in every trivia, karaoke, and dancing night. I could never forget that amazing mother-daughter trip.

Reality resumed as soon as we got home and on October 30th, 2017, Dr. McGill placed a free-flowing shunt with no valve in my abdomen. The surgery was successful. Even though he had no choice, I will always hate that McGill did that shunt because my fears were correct. One uplifting memory from that day is the flowers that my sister Olivia sent me with a card that read *Kick this shunt's ass. Love you bunches*. I'll always remember and cherish that card. (P.S. I still have it.)

2017 quickly flowed into 2018 and I was splitting my time between bible study, family, managing my health, and working at a retirement home. I was a med tech at a local retirement home for a couple of years and I loved working the peaceful night shifts. I had struggled to find an employer who wouldn't fire me for missing work due to surgeries, but this boss was brilliant. I also worked with a lovely med tech named Karissa who I would hang out with after work and goof off with on breaks. I remember once we were put under investigation by the police for missing morphine- it wasn't us though!

In January, I was getting closer to Aaron. Whenever bible study was at his house, he would ask me to come early so I could cut his hair. I was by no means a hairdresser and I didn't realize that he only asked because he had a huge crush on me. By the end of the month, brain pressure symptoms were getting worse again but that would have to wait because my long-awaited Make-A-Wish trip was finally happening. A limo picked up my mom, stepdad, Emilie, and me on February 23rd at around 3 am and there were even fancy champagne glasses with non-alcoholic wine. We took a flight out of Eugene, stopped in Portland, and continued on to Florida. On the plane, we wore bright blue Make-A-Wish t-shirts and one of the lovely pilots gave me a gift. The cruise started in Florida and then took us to St Maarten, Puerto Rico, and Haiti. We spent an entire day in St Maarten on a private beach and because we were with Make-A-Wish, people brought us free drinks, fruit, and snacks all day long. It was a fabulous experience, and the views were beautiful especially the magnificently blue ocean. In Puerto Rico, my mom and stepdad went on an ATV day trip while Emilie and I hung out with the executive chef from our ship who showed us around, took us to get some delicious crab and went shopping. Haiti was my favorite place. The people were so friendly, the water was crystal clear so we could see every tiny creature on the seabed, and Emilie and I took the longest zipline over the ocean. Emmie was super excited about the zipline until we reached the top of the steps and she wanted to go back. I said she wasn't allowed- she probably was, however, I wasn't going to let her wimp out. So, side by side we flew high above the ocean and she deafened me with her screams, but it was beautiful. We could see all of Haiti with its blossoming colors and tiny people going about their days as if nobody was watching them from the sky. After we made it to the bottom of the mountain of steps, Emilie asked to go again and I said no... once was plenty!

On the cruising days, we had shows and all sorts of fun stuff to do. My mom and I did all the trivia games, just like on our first cruise. We still got special treatment, like the best seats for every show, meet and greets with the cast, and private tours of the kitchen, captain's deck, jail and the morgue. I remember that the morgue could fit up to 25 people... that doesn't spring to mind with the word 'cruise', but I guess they've got to have one. Seeing the captain's deck was fascinating. The captain told me to press a button, so I did but I didn't let go.

With a furrowed brow he said, 'Don't you hear that?!' and I replied 'Nope'.

Then he said 'Okay, okay, let go! That's the horn!' and I let go, laughing.

It was just my mom and me, so only we knew the hilarious expression of irritation on his face. While we did that, Emilie and my stepdad were doing a surfing activity that Emmie loved and I did not. That entire trip was paid for by Make-A-Wish and it was the most relaxing break without having to worry about the costs. That charity gave our family such a cherished memory so I can never pass up donating towards another family's happiness now.

After our wonderful cruise, normality resumed once again, and on March 13th, I got my LP shunt replaced. I had this awful pain in my abdomen, and I just knew it was that shunt already causing trouble. The X-ray showed that the entire free-floating tube had fallen from my spine into my pelvis. Dr. McGill opened me up, put it back, and closed me up again. On the 17th, I ended up back in hospital because the suture on my spine opened up at the top. Once the suture was closed, the problems were fixed...briefly.

My mom had started working with Aaron and I would drop into his office to see her all the time- always in my baggy scrubs after work. One time, I went into the office wearing normal, fitted clothes and Aaron suddenly perked up like a cat who heard 'treats'. The office was tiny, and I had to walk past Aaron's desk to get to my mom's.

After I kissed my mom goodbye, I was squeezing past Aaron's desk, and he joked 'Where's mine?'

I aimed for his forehead, but he lifted his head, so I pushed it back down, gave him a timid peck on the forehead, and rushed out of the office. I texted 'Were you gonna kiss me?' He responded with, 'Duh!'. I typed 'We should set a date first' and he replied with that day's date.

The next day at the office, I kissed him goodbye on the lips and whispered, 'I owed you that'.

Our first date was after work on April 27th, 2018. After so many bible study meetups, we already felt at home with each other, so it was a relaxed first date. Aaron bought us Café Yumm without knowing I hated that kind of food. After that little hiccup, we went for a sunny spring walk in the park and saw a huge salamander, and the rest is history.

Less than two months into dating Aaron, my LP shunt decided to misbehave. At the beginning of June, I had abdominal pain and high-pressure symptoms, but Dr. McGill was adamant that it couldn't be broken again. That was one doctor who would dismiss me, even if Aaron came to the appointment with me, and it was frustrating to feel unheard about something so serious. However, the scans proved that I was right and that it had fallen into my pelvis again. Dr. McGill put it back in its place, but the same thing happened again in July, and I needed surgery twice within one week. On July 5th, I had a raging fever, and my side was swollen where the shunt tubing was. I went to Corvallis Hospital in an ambulance and had emergency surgery where they took the infected tubing out, cleaned the infection, and replaced the entire shunt. I was on antibiotics for the infection and recovery was terrible. Five days later, the tubing fell into my pelvis again! So, after the fourth revision, Dr. McGill finally decided to stitch the tube into my spine so that it could no longer fall.

The next month, it was the VP shunt's turn to cause trouble. I thought my summer couldn't get much worse, but it did. It really did. On August 29th, Dr. McGill did a VP shunt revision.

The surgeon told my mom, 'Elise is playing a really high-stakes poker game here.'

Those were frightening words from a neurosurgeon and my mom seemed worried when she told me about it.

I replied, 'I'm really good at poker, Mom', kissed her, and was rolled away to the chilly operating room again.

During that surgery, Dr. McGill tried to pull the old catheter out, which caused a bleed on the brain. He quickly cleaned up the bleed and left it alone, placing a new catheter in the second to last possible ventricle. Afterward, he was honest about his mistake to Aaron and my mom. He said it should be fine but the next day, we discovered that my entire left side was numb, and I couldn't walk. After one shunt revision after another, a TIA was the rotten cherry on top. I had to stay at a rehab facility for a month to learn how to use my left side again. The consequence of that surgery was possibly my most difficult hurdle yet, but I was just lucky to be alive. Well, I *am* really good at poker.

A rehab facility was the worst place to recover after surgery; I just wanted to be at home. My family and Aaron visited every night which made it a little easier. A bunch of people would drop by most days, and my hairdresser would come to wash my hair with proper shampoo because the facility wasn't too concerned about hair care. The first Physical Therapist I had was an awful man who was more suited to the role of a drill sergeant. He told me to walk down the hallway and I tried so hard to do it, but I just couldn't. I was crying with pain and frustration while dragging myself at a snail's pace down that hallway.

My mom kept shouting 'Stop, she can't do it!' but he continued yelling at me.

After being belittled for a few minutes, my body couldn't do it anymore and I hit the cold tiles hard. I felt like an empty shell of a human at that moment.

He shouted, 'Get up and go again'.

My mom stormed up to him and yelled, 'No! Go and get me another member of staff, now!'.

The man just stood there as she struggled to get me off the floor and into my wheelchair. Once I was in the chair, she found the person in charge and complained. Yet, this guy continued to yell at me throughout the few other sessions that I was forced to share with him. Eventually, they switched him to a lovely young woman with beautiful long black hair who understood that everybody has limits.

Aaron says that the hardest part to watch was the occupational therapy sessions. My occupational therapist was a sweet older lady, and she would fill a bowl with basic, everyday objects and then cover them in rice. I closed my eyes, dug around, and held an object that I knew the feeling of in my left hand but when she asked what it was, I couldn't tell her. My brain wouldn't communicate with my hand, and it felt like little pieces of my mind had crumbled into nothing. Every time Aaron watched this, his eyes filled with tears because he felt so helpless. Every day of that recovery was dehumanizing in a hundred different ways, and it was a prolonged process. It took the entire month before I was even close to getting the right answer during that activity.

Most of the people in the facility were much older than me, but I noticed one young guy during mealtimes. I also noticed his teardrop tattoos.

After one week of noticing each other, he knocked on my open door and asked, 'What are you doing here? You're young'.

I said, 'So are you.'

Liam explained that he also had a TIA, but it was caused by fighting. He could still walk though. I asked about his teardrop tattoos, pretending that I didn't know their meaning.

He fumbled, 'I did some bad stuff.'

I asked what and he said 'I killed a few people to defend myself... and my fight was in prison. I'll be going back there soon.'

I called him stupid, and he chuckled, 'You're blunt aren't you?'

I hear that a lot. There were no guards at the facility, but there was always a nurse or two keeping a close eye on him. It turned out that he had a little son and after I found that out, I would often tell him how stupid he was for wasting his life along with ruining his son's. He always said my words were blunt, but he never disagreed with them.

I remember that he wore his trousers low and one time my mom saw it and said, 'Pull those up, I can see your panties'.

Liam never wore them low down after that. We grew close and he would always check up on me and get whatever I needed.

The first time I invited Liam to play games with my family, Aaron waited until he couldn't hear us before whispering, 'Elise, he's from prison, and those tattoos... be careful!'.

I teased him saying, 'No, really?', but after they hung out together Aaron agreed that he was a nice guy.

By the end of our time together, Liam had an altered perspective on life. He was more positive and determined to improve his life after his release. I guess all it took was a random blunt woman telling him to stop wasting his life and prioritize his kid for that to become a possibility. I also told him to cover up those tattoos because they ruined his good looks and told the world who he used to be. He thought that was a good idea. We lost touch, but wherever he is now, I hope he's with his son and on a better path.

My favorite memory from that awful month was probably Aaron and Oreo. Now and then, Aaron was allowed to take me on a short drive, and he knew how much I missed my little cat Oreo. She was the sweetest most protective pet, and I knew she would be missing me too. Aaron bundled her into her cat carrier before visiting me so that I could cuddle her while we ate lunch in the car. That was a savored moment. I had Oreo for sixteen years and we grew up together. When I was a toddler, I used to suck my thumb with one hand and hold her paw with the other while she copied me by licking her spare paw. While I was in rehab, my mom, and our vet Rachel, who I was friends with, discovered that Oero had two different types of cancer. I barely saw her while I was there, so they decided not to tell me. Not long after I got home, I took Oreo to Rachel because she didn't seem like herself at all. Rachel reassured me that it was just old age and then called my mom saying that they needed to tell me the truth. In October, my mom told me how sick Oreo was because I was finally well enough to hear the truth. I was outraged that they kept it from me. I never thought myself too unwell to handle things and I would have ended her suffering months ago. Putting her down was devastating because I lost my childhood best friend, but I'll always remember the beautiful memories she gave me, like when she brightened up rehab.

When I got home from the rehab facility, I had to stay downstairs because walking was still new and exhausting. At the next appointment, Dr. McGill retracted his admittance of causing a brain bleed. He claimed that I never had one. McGill said this to the people he had been honest with just weeks before. My eye doctor saw proof of the TIA and imaging reports still show evidence of it, so there was no foundation for his lie. The frustrating part was that I wasn't even mad because I knew the risks of brain surgery and I was just grateful that someone was still willing to perform them on me. As soon as McGill started lying, I had a feeling that he was going to dump me out of fear of getting sued. I remember crying with Aaron in the McDonald's parking lot because I didn't know what to do if McGill dumped me.

On Christmas Eve that year, I got the dreaded MyChart message from McGill, except it said that he was retiring. There was another girl with IIH that I knew from McGill's waiting room, and I asked her if she was still seeing him and of course, she was. So, I was back to square one of finding another neurosurgeon.

Even though I had a stroke, lost my cat, and ended up with no neurosurgeon, 2018 still holds some wonderful memories. Before Christmas, Emilie, Aaron, and I went camping in Mount Hood. We took Aaron's trailer and went sledding, had snowball fights, made smores, and took a train to the top of the mountain. We also went swimming and met a man who looked identical to Dwayne 'the Rock' Johnson. Of course, we knew it wasn't him, but we kept the joke alive and to this day we reminisce about playing with the Rock and his kids... or pebbles. That Christmas, Aaron presented me with the most fabulous gift. My family loves to play Monopoly, and Aaron always wins, so he handmade a huge Monopoly board specifically catered to all things Elise. It included *pay Elise's medical bills*, *get a spinal tap*, *get a CAT scan,* etc. Despite McGill's letdown, Aaron made that Christmas special.

Chapter Seven

A t the start of January 2019, my mom found another neuro-surgeon. She asked an IIH group again and found the highly recommended Dr. D, then she sent him daily letters until he accepted a consultation.

During that meeting, he said 'I read all of your files... you're very complicated. You've had so many surgeries because shunts are not meant for you.'

I have been told it's like putting Ford parts in a Ferrari. Eventually, he said that he would take me on but only for two surgeries. I teared up at that because I knew he would drop me pretty soon if that were the case.

So, I said 'I will get a contract written up that guarantees myself or my family will never sue you. But I need you to do as many surgeries as it takes to keep me alive. We know the risks so if the opposite happens, my family will not sue you.'

He saw my desperation and said no to the contract, but still agreed to my request. That's how I got the wonderful neurosurgeon that I have today.

Every year, Aaron's friends go snow camping... except they rent a house so it's not camping. I had gotten to know all of his friends pretty well, so I was invited that year. On January 18th, we traveled to Bend,

Oregon. We were given the enormous master bedroom that even had a jacuzzi in it. Unfortunately, we only got to enjoy it for one night because, by the next day, I had a raging fever, tachycardia, and terrible head pain. Aaron and his friend Jamie took me to St. Charles Hospital where they did a CT scan. The doctor said, 'Her hydrocephalus is fine.'

Aaron replied, 'But she doesn't have that.'

The doctor then claimed that hydrocephalus is the only reason people get shunts. Aaron was appalled that he had to, but he explained IIH and told her to do an MRI then adjust my shunt afterwards. The doctor agreed but when Aaron asked if they had the correct machine to adjust my valve, she said no but was planning to do the MRI anyway. I am so glad that while I was barely conscious, Aaron was there to furiously insist that she call Dr. D because she clearly had no idea what she was doing. She hesitantly called Dr. D, and he asked St Charles Hospital to transfer me over to him. The doctor initially refused but after Dr. D convinced her, we were on a 'non-emergency ambulance' for about four hours to Portland. The change in altitude traveling from Bend to Portland twice in two days made things much worse because altitude changes affect brain pressure. When we got to Dr. D, he found that the issue was a serious infection.

Once I was better, in February, Aaron and I went camping on the coast in Newport. This was something that we adored doing. We would both work all week, so most weekends we would get in the RV and spend our spare time at the beach. It would either be Lincoln City, Florence, or Newport. We would walk on the beach for hours, explore the local areas, get fish sticks and clam chowder at Mo's, and then either watch TV in the RV or build a campfire. Thrift stores always lured us in (well, me...), and Aaron would embarrass me by playing one of the two songs he knew on any piano he could find. One time, we found a piano that you played by using your feet and he was so badly uncoordinated that it was hilarious. That month, Aaron sold his business that he had owned for most of his life and chose propane truck driving so that he could see more of Oregon's countryside. One time, he was sent to a conference in Bend, and I went with him. We stayed in the old mill district and had dinner at a lovely little restaurant called Anthony's. I had gotten lost multiple times while Aaron worked, and I remember saying how much I hated that confusing place. We had no idea that a couple of years later, we would settle down there, become regulars at Anthony's, and have to use a GPS forever.

In April, we went camping in Florence and I wanted to get dinner somewhere new. There was a casino that I wanted to dine at, but I wasn't 21 yet. Aaron is such a stickler for rules that it took a while to convince him. We got in without getting carded, but he still avoided eye contact like a nervous criminal. We didn't play the slots or drink, we just got food, so it was completely harmless. Aaron was so stressed that someone would ask my age that he even refused to take a selfie because it was 'proof'.

I laughed, 'You're worried someone will recognize this random casino from the blank wall behind us?'

When we got back in the car I teased, 'Oh no, Aaron, do you hear sirens?'

He was so nervous that someone would find out about our heinous crime. It's published now, sorry hubby.

At the end of April, we visited Astoria, Oregon, which was pretty far from us. Aaron and I explored Fort Stevens, the Lewis and Clark National Historical Park, and saw the Astoria Column. We also raced each other at a kid's funfair. I fitted in the tiny car, but Aaron's feet were in his chest, so I won. In Astoria, we passed a sign that said, 'Elsie Street' and medical professionals have always mistaken my name for

Elsie, so obviously I took a picture with it. Overall, that was one of my favorite camping trips.

At this point in life, Aaron and I were always on the go between working and enjoying life together. At the time, I was working as one of two caregivers for a family with two disabled children. It was a hectic but rewarding job. In March 2019, we took the two children and Emilie on a day trip to a safari park. The kids loved it. Ostriches ate out of their hands, and the elephants painted pictures for the kids with their trunks.

In May, the whole family went to a tulip festival. I took a photo of my mom pretending to cut the tulips. This was an inside joke because when she was young, she cut all of my Nana's prized tulips and brought them to her as a gift. Not long after that was Mother's Day. Aaron and I took our moms out to lunch at a beautiful woodland eatery. We sat under warm spring sunbeams while our moms began their usual discussion about marriage.

It went something like, 'Y'all need to get married! This place is so cute... it would be perfect for your wedding.'

We weren't ready to get married yet and life was far too busy. We got annoyed because this conversation was a regular occurrence, and our moms would team up against us. Although ironically, we did get married there.

At the end of May, my mom and I went to Seattle because my ophthalmologist, Dr. Ambiti, suggested a specialist who could discuss doing ONSF. This is a procedure called optic nerve sheath decompression which relieves papilledema caused by raised brain pressure. Papilledema is something that I don't usually get, but it makes doctors take IIH much more seriously because it's undeniable proof that there is an issue. The specialist thought that the next shunt surgery would likely fix the papilledema, so they agreed not to do it yet. My mom suggested that I get it done anyway because it was affecting my vision. I said no because papilledema could be evidence of any underlying issue that would otherwise go unnoticed. Dr. Ambiti recently asked if I wanted to get it done, but I still don't because it's the only thing that proves deterioration and ensures fast-paced help when I need it. Even though I decided against ONSF, Mom and I stayed at a nice hotel and enjoyed varenyky at a Ukrainian restaurant, so Seattle wasn't a wasted trip.

The spring of 2019 had been filled with delightful memories and minimal hospital visits, but I knew that sooner or later that was going to change.

Chapter Eight

At the start of June, I met with Dr. D's physician's assistant, Kareen, because I knew something was wrong with the VP shunt. My vision and hearing were both going, and the head pain was terrible. The hospital did an X-ray, CT scan, and an MRI, but everything came back normal. I begged Kareen to keep trying to figure out what was wrong, so she ordered a 'shunt-o-gram'. This is where they inject a contrast dye into the shunt valve and track how it flows through the tubing to detect any blockages or issues. On the second day of tests, they did the shunt-o-gram. The nurse injected the dye and said it would take a few minutes to go through.

I replied, 'It won't.'

We waited for at least two hours, but the dye hadn't moved. The nurse called Kareen, who said I needed to walk for 20 minutes to make the dye move.

I said, 'Okay' and walked around the corridors for a while.

They looked for the dye with the imaging machine again, but still nothing. By this point, it was nearly four hours since my appointment started and the patients after me were piling up in the waiting room.

The nurse called Kareen again and she said I had to go and sit down for an hour while they saw some of the other patients and then they would try one more time.

I said, 'Okay' and sat for an hour, with awful pressure from the dye just sitting there.

Five hours after it was injected, they looked for the dye again, but it still hadn't moved. This time, Kareen came down to the room.

She was fed up with me messing up her workday and said in a snooty, sarcastic voice, 'Well, you're really atypical aren't you?'

'I told you it was broken,' I replied.

We're friends now and she's still mortified that she said that to me. I found it hilarious because obviously, I understood her frustration.

After that test, Kareen let Dr. D know that all four components of the valve seemed to be broken and they scheduled surgery. I had to stay at a hotel the night before the shunt-o-gram and I was planning to go home that day, but it was unsafe to drive home with the head pain, so I stayed another night.

On June 12th, I had revision surgery to replace the valve and tubing. Before the surgery, Dr. D used little donut-shaped stickers to map areas of my brain and my entire forehead puffed up with donut-shaped rashes that looked like some kind of plague. Turns out I was just allergic to Mastisol, the glue they used. For this surgery, they did the usual head incision and four incisions in my abdomen to move the tubing but then an extra horseshoe incision in a painful spot at the back of my head.

This surgery was the last one until 2021 and I was very thankful for the break, even though it came with side effects.

I finally turned 21 on July 14th, 2019, and I had just healed from the last surgery. My favorite gift was a tattoo on my leg that says, 'You are my sunshine'. That one was for my Nana.

My stepdad and Aaron insisted on taking me out for my first drink at the stroke of midnight on my birthday.

After that first drink I said, 'Okay, we can go home now.'

I wasn't a big fan of drinking then, and even now, I only drink occasionally. Aaron's mom's retirement party was on my birthday, and it was at a Beaver's baseball game in Corvallis.

I'd never been to a sports game, and I remember Aaron asking, 'Do you know what's happening... it looks like you're enjoying it?'

I said, 'I don't know what's happening, but I love the tight little pants.'

After that, my family arranged a big party for me at Buffalo Wild Wings. It was a lovely celebration with everyone, and people gave speeches and gave me beautiful presents. After the party, my friends took me to a proper bar because they wanted me to get drunk. That didn't happen, but I did have a great night with them and Aaron. Birthdays never felt important, but now that I've surpassed the age I was supposed to die, they feel like a gift.

A couple of days after my birthday, we went to Aaron's huge family reunion. There were what felt like 100 people there and as an introvert, it was nice but overwhelming. Aaron is an extrovert, so he disappears into a crowd, while I like to stand on the sidelines. I only became introverted after I got ill because people have a habit of presenting me to a group with, 'This is Elise, she has a rare illness!'

At the end of July, Aaron and I went to Lane County Fair. I had never been to a big county fair before, but I knew that I wasn't allowed on most of the rides due to the gravitational changes. We petted the pigs, walked through the enchanting butterfly exhibit, and went on the Ferris wheel because it was too slow to make me sick. I begged Aaron to go on a couple of big rides so I could live vicariously through him, but he hates rides, so he took some convincing. He went on one that looked pretty tame, but I saw the panic set into his eyes as it sped up and began throwing him around. He got off the ride with a green tinge and refused to go on another one ever again. We also got a caricature done in which Aaron was turned into this big goon while I was a cute little doll. He wasn't ecstatic about that either, but I liked it. Something finally went his way when we were pulled up on stage for a magic trick and Aaron won by picking the Queen card.

He presented it to me with 'because you're my queen' and it's lived in my purse ever since.

Things were still going relevantly smoothly since my last revision, which I was grateful for because we had a 7-day Alaskan cruise booked for the whole family. At the beginning of September, Aaron, myself, my mom, Steve, Emilie, Olivia, my hairdresser friend Ashley, and her little son Zi all met up in Washington to go on our cruise. We're very close with Ashley and her son was always my little Valentine. He was even our ring bearer at the wedding, and he was adorably furious about losing me to Aaron. The night before departure, we all had dinner at a Mexican restaurant, and it was the first time Aaron was meeting my sister Olivia because she still lived in Wyoming.

Aaron went to hug Olivia, but she put her hand up and said, 'It's nice to meet you. Don't touch me though.'

I thought *here we go* because my sister has always been unpredictable. They didn't talk for the entire meal, and I could feel the discomfort radiating from Aaron. When we got to our hotel room, he asked me what that was and I had to explain that it was generally just Olivia. My sister and I are total opposites in most aspects but particularly in that I like people and she does not.

The next day when we boarded the cruise ship, my mom gave Aaron and me matching baseball caps labeled 'Captain' and 'First Mate'. As we've established, my mom and Aaron are best friends, so he got the 'Captain' one. The first night on the ship was formal dress and I had this gorgeous floor-length teal dress, but I realized that I had forgotten to pack the matching shoes. Normally I wouldn't care at all, but with Olivia there, I knew there would be comments made if my outfit wasn't perfect. After about 45 minutes of panicking about shoes, Aaron convinced me that the black ones I had would be fine because you could barely see them under the dress.

We met up with everybody in the dining room and the first thing I heard was 'Your shoes don't match.'

I replied, 'Thank you' and sat down with a ruined mood and a desire for pajamas and solitude.

My mom forced us to have a photo together, but I felt so self-conscious that my smile wasn't the most convincing. Olivia refused to have a photo with Aaron, so my mom happily took a bunch of herself and him. When we got back to our room, it took me 0.5 seconds to get into my pajamas and wipe my face off. I told Aaron I was already over the trip, so we decided to avoid Olivia and just enjoy ourselves. So, we saw the whole ship from the skylight and Aaron took Emilie on the skydiving simulator where their cheeks flapped in the wind like chipmunks.

My mom and I did a trivia night where they had dollar mimosas and I asked her, 'How many can we carry?'

She said, 'Well we have ten fingers each.'

We both knocked on our doors with our feet and Aaron opened ours to me balancing ten wobbly mimosas. The next day Emilie wanted to go on the bumper cars so Aaron, Steve, Emilie, and I went on them and all of us adults got off them feeling like we had whiplash. Emilie wanted to go again so we had to explain that after a certain age, bumper cars just feel like a million tiny car accidents.

That night was another formal evening and we all met up in the huge, dazzling dining room. While enjoying a delicious dinner, we somehow got onto my mom's favorite topic- Aaron and I getting married. We still didn't feel ready for marriage, but maybe we were getting closer.

During the discussion, Olivia blurted out, 'Aaron, if you're going to marry Elise, you'd better ask my dad for permission.'

The table fell silent, and Aaron said, 'Well, I don't think I need any permission other than Elise's but if I was going to ask anyone, it would probably be Steve.'

Olivia turned a violent shade of red and began to rage in front of about 500 finely dressed people. My mom told her to stop because she agreed that Aaron could do whatever he wanted. At that point, Olivia stood up, spilled her drink all over the tablecloth, and stormed out. Aaron apologized to everyone, but my mom reassured him that none of it was his fault before she left to find Olivia. The rest of us sat there with hundreds of eyes fixed on us and icy silence, other than the occasional scraping of cutlery. Even though I wanted to evaporate right out of my fancy dress, I was impressed with how Aaron won that battle.

That night solidified the original plan to keep to ourselves, so we began treating it more like a romantic cruise for two. On September 8th, we stopped in Juno for our first shore day. Ziplining is one activity that I'm definitely not supposed to do but it's one that I adore and will always do. Life's too short to follow all the rules all the time. So, Aaron and I ziplined through the Alaskan forest and it was beautiful. Then we went hiking, saw a glacier, and even tried our hand at axe throwing... that's one skill we won't be adding to our resumes. The next day, we visited Skagway and took a bus tour with my mom and Steve. We learned about a murderer who had killed people in Oregon, fled to Alaska, gained a position of power, and then got caught. I also remember an Alaskan crab leg restaurant with a big crab on the front that used to be an old brothel and it said 'Yes, we have crabs.' That was perfect.

The next day was an at-sea day and Aaron, and I watched a quiz game about marriage in which the younger couples knew nothing about each other and the older couples got every question right. One couple were both detectives yet neither could remember what the other was wearing.

When the older couple were asked, the husband said, 'How would I know? She's already changed twice today!'

After that show, there was a hypnotist and Aaron tried to convince me that it was real, but we ran into the participants afterward and they told us they were acting. Aaron will never stop hearing that I was right. We also went to an enchanting *Alice in Wonderland*-themed restaurant. The chairs had white rabbit ears or checkerboard patterns and the dining room was a sea of beautiful blues, purples, and reds with cascading chandeliers. My favorite part was the mystical mushroom garden dessert which used mousse, meringue, and sorbet to create little mushrooms sprouting out of soil and grass. It was magical.

The final fun day was a trip to Victoria, British Columbia. Emilie hung out with Zi and Ashley while Mom, Steve, Aaron, and I explored the drizzly town with our umbrellas. We saw the magnificent castle with turquoise tips and walked through a garden that bloomed the most vividly colored roses I had ever seen. We were shameless tourists, even taking photos in a random hotel bathroom because it had a huge, embellished vanity mirror. After the explosive dinner was forgotten, that trip became one of the most wonderful we've ever been on.

The rest of that year was very relaxed compared to my version of normality, and it was bliss. However, on October 20th, we lost my lovely Aunt Tammy. Aunt Tammy was my mom's only sister and she lived in Deer Park, Texas with my cousins Jacob and Zac. I was never very close to her while growing up, but when I got sick, we found that we had a lot more to bond over. She was a different kind of sick because she battled with cancer but with very few unwell people in the family, we found an understanding within each other. We began calling each other when one of us was in the hospital and checking in often. It was kind of like having a sick buddy. I'll always remember when she came to stay with us, and we took her to the coast. I loved getting to see her in person.

We got the phone call about her passing while out to dinner and my mom went into complete denial at first. In Texas, a paramedic alone can't pronounce a person deceased because the hospital has to confirm it. So, when Jacob said that they had taken her to the hospital in an ambulance, my mom hoped that she would still be alive, even though they knew that wasn't the case. My mom was distraught, so I immediately flew with her to Texas and the rest of the family followed a few days later.

When we were kids, Jacob was closer to Olivia so I felt excluded, and when I got sick, he was one of the many people who avoided talking to me completely. I just assumed people did that because they didn't know what to say but that didn't make it feel any better. When it was just me and him at Aunt Tammy's house after her passing, he tried to connect with me again.

He asked, 'Why don't we talk anymore?'

I said, 'Because you all stopped talking to me when I got sick.'

He thought about it for a minute and then apologized. He spent the next few days trying to reconnect with me and we bonded over old photos and grief.

Zac moved out to Oregon in December and Jacob followed not long afterward, which was amazing for our growing friendship.

Chapter Nine

2020 was a difficult year for people all over the world and for a few unexpected reasons, it was an unusual year for me too.

At the beginning of the summer, Aaron was offered a job in a different state, and he was desperate to accept it. He asked if I would move away with him, but I wasn't going to live with a partner unless we were married. At that point, neither of us felt completely ready for marriage but I knew that I wanted to marry him soon, just not for this reason.

So, we parted ways and Aaron moved away while I moved out to get some more independence. Marriage wasn't right for us at that moment in time and we both needed to be apart to grow and discover what we did and didn't want out of life. Despite my devastation, Jacob and I found a lovely apartment to share and were excited to make up for lost time. On July 3rd, 2020, I moved in with Jacob and we were like a couple of kids. He would bring home the weirdest things for me to bake which were usually gross. He would also build days' worth of Lego that my cat would destroy in seconds. My cat Mercury loved to watch him gaming on his computer. As much as she enjoyed destroying his things, she loved him, so she became more like a shared cat than my own. After Jacob spent hours teaching me to play Halo, my gaming sessions would always end with him shouting, 'No, you have to shoot them! Wait, no...and you died.' Living with Jacob felt like having a brother and I adored it.

One memory that we still joke about today is feet pics. It was the first time I had been single in my adult life, and I was blissfully unaware of how many feet pic requests single women get. I decided to have a little fun and play along when I got those requests.

I would say that my feet were super cute with fresh pedicures and then run downstairs shouting, 'Jacob, some guy offered me $50 for my feet pics, give me your feet now!'.

After sending the creeps a photo of Jacob's big manly feet I asked, 'You want my Venmo now?'

We still randomly text each other, 'Feet pics?' to reminisce about our time living together.

A few weeks later, I got a text from Aaron asking if we could meet.

It turns out that Aaron asked his mom if he should marry me and she said, 'You'd be an idiot not to.'

When we split up, his mom and I wanted to stay friends but I couldn't be friends with Aaron when I still loved him, so he said that it was okay for us two to keep in touch. I was very grateful for her little speech that solidified his decision to text me.

On October 3rd, we were hiking and Aaron asked me to be his girlfriend again.

'I don't know, I need to think about it', I answered.

We had agreed to spend the day together and it was still early when he stood on top of that mountain looking helplessly miserable at my response. Around 6 pm, we grabbed dinner at a diner, and I was carefully watching him eat his food.

He said, 'This is good.'

After a few seconds, I shouted, 'Yes!'

He looked up, startled, and replied, 'Yes... this food is good?'

I laughed, 'Yes, I'll date you again!'

Coincidentally, I did exactly what his mom did to his dad. She left him hanging for hours after the important question before saying yes. At least I followed tradition.

Those couple of months apart made Aaron and I remember why we chose each other in the first place. We needed to grow a little by ourselves before we could keep growing together.

When Aaron and I first got back in touch in September, I was starting to wake up every morning with headaches in the back of my head. It was unusual so I assumed it was low brain pressure and tried an energy drink, which helped. As it continued, I got imaging done and it showed mild Chiari. Dr. D was uncomfortable with performing Chiari surgery on me, so he was relieved that it was mild enough to just monitor. However, it gradually got worse over the next three months.

The pain started to become an issue every time I stood up. I started to miss work and couldn't drive because sitting upright in the car became too painful. Nothing would help except for energy drinks, and they only caused very slight relief. When Steve saw how many I had in the fridge, he was so concerned about my heart. I remember saying that if my heart was the thing that took me out, God would have to send me back down because, after everything I'd been through, I was not going to accept that.

Jacob was a godsend because whenever he was home, he would keep me company while I was bored from having to lie down all the time. We watched so many kid's movies together, including all of the Shrek movies. One time, I was taking a bath, and out of nowhere, my head started hurting so intensely. I tried to stand up to get out, but I couldn't do it, so I had to call for Jacob. He closed his eyes and wrapped two towels around me before getting me into bed.

A similar thing happened when Emilie came for a sleepover. The pain always got worse by the evening but usually, I could get through it. I had bought an Xbox for Emilie and me to play on, and she was getting it ready for a gaming night. I was standing in the bathroom and suddenly I couldn't stand up anymore. Emilie found me lying on the floor crying. She got Jacob and he managed to get me into bed. It got to the point where he was doing this constantly and then getting everything for me so that I wouldn't have to stand up. He would take me to all of my appointments by helping me to the car, driving me, and then helping me in and out of the appointments, even if that meant carrying me. He was truly a godsend and I'm so grateful for everything he did.

I had more imaging done in December and got a call from Dr. D quite late in the evening. He told me that the Chiari had deteriorated from a small herniation to an extremely dangerous one. My brain was falling so far down that it was beginning to collapse my brain stem. My LP shunt had caused it. It was pulling too much fluid down and it had started to pull my brain down at an increasingly rapid rate. If it had been left much longer, it would have killed me. Dr. D said that it had to be fixed as soon as possible and it was going to be an incredibly advanced and high-risk surgery. He had to check if I wanted to do it after learning about the risk.

I asked, 'What other choices do I have?' because there were none.

He told me that they would be using a cow membrane to keep my brain hoisted up in place.

For months after that surgery, we often made cow jokes and my mom's favorite was 'You're being so mooody'.

On January 11th, 2021, I had the Chiari Malformation surgery. Everybody came for this one, even my dad. However, COVID restrictions meant that only one person could come in with me. It had always been my mom, then my mom and Aaron but from then onwards it became just Aaron.

For typical Chiari surgery, they only remove the top skull flap, but my brain was herniating so deeply that they also had to remove the middle of the top two vertebrae. Even though they pulled my brain back up, it can take about a year for the swelling to shrink down into place properly. After the surgery, my body and shunts needed some time to learn how to behave normally again and there was too much CSF fluid so, they did an external shunt. CSF flows down your spine, so, similarly to where they place a lumbar puncture needle, they insert a plastic tube to drain the excess fluid. The tube came out of my back and connected to a bag that was hung up next to me. The nurses had to release the fluid every fifteen minutes and I would sit there sobbing every time. It was the most painful experience and the pain shot from my head to my toes, radiating agony throughout my body. It should never hurt that much, so Dr. D came to observe and figured out that a nerve must have been getting sucked into the tube every time they released the fluid. They pulled the tube down, hoping to avoid the nerve but that didn't help for very long. Dr. D agreed that the nurses could stretch the 15 minutes into 30 minutes because they felt awful frequently causing such agony. After five days, Dr. D allowed them to take the tube out. Even that was painful, as it felt like it was ripped out. Aaron still remembers seeing me in that pain, but he had learned by that point that if something wouldn't typically go wrong, it would for me.

On January 16th, I finally got to go home. Emilie came back to the apartment because she wanted to help Jacob look after me. My mom and Emilie had been shoved out of the way due to pandemic restrictions, so she was glad to come home with me. I wasn't allowed to do anything for weeks after this surgery. This one was different because I was missing parts of my neck so there are rules even to this day, for example, I can't get my hair washed in a hairdresser's chair because the bowl presses on the surgery area. After six weeks, I had to start physical therapy to learn how to move my neck properly and where I could or couldn't touch it. Jacob was back to getting me everything I needed and helping me around the house. Whenever he was working, my mom would come and take over. They made a great team.

On January 23rd, Debbie, a friend from church brought over candies and a fabulous big blue 'get well soon' balloon. Jacob helped me down onto the floor and we sat opposite each other with Mercury and the balloon in the middle. For some reason, Mercury was terrified of it, so we started batting it back and forth towards her. After a while of teasing her, Jacob put it out of the way in my bedroom. That night, she refused to come into my room for cuddles until Jacob moved the balloon. He put it in my closet but then she sat and watched the closet door, anxiously waiting for it to pop out. Eventually, she came to bed and forgot about it but the next morning when she followed me into my closet, she shot out of there like a roadrunner. I've never been able to have balloons in my house since then.

After the incisions healed, I got mandala designs shaved into the tiny bit of hair I had on the back of my head. The hospital had pretty much given me an undercut, so I just embraced it.

That was a complex surgery, but I had been through much worse, and I was just relieved to have my brain back where it belongs.

I got the most amazing post-surgery gift from Jacob. This one was special because anyone who knows me knows that I adore penguins. So, Jacob adopted an emperor penguin in my name and surprised me with the certificate and a penguin plushie. I love knowing that my little penguin is still out there in the snow somewhere.

A month later, I was doing much better. For Valentine's Day, Aaron surprised me with a short trip to Eugene. When we arrived, there was a beautiful old-fashioned bungalow ready for us, and inside, Aaron had prepared a planner with a very detailed itinerary for our trip. Our room had a huge jacuzzi, which made up for the fancy jacuzzi we missed out on in January 2019. There was a sign that said 'Don't put bubbles in the tub' but we didn't notice that until we had bubble beards. The owners lived on-site in a blue house with white trim, and there was a fabulous mini version of the house outside for their Bengal cat. That trip was a wonderful way to ease me back into a life that isn't based on bed rest.

Chapter Nine

At the beginning of 2021, Aaron was living in Pacific City for work. It was under two hours away, so we didn't mind traveling to see each other. On March 22nd, I visited him for a few days. At first, we hung out at the beach, and I played with his cat Boy Kitty. He's our cat now. On the 24th, we went for a drive and Aaron kept saying he wanted to show me something. He drove us up a hill by the coast and stopped outside of some gorgeous houses to ask me if I could imagine living around there.

It was beautiful, so I said 'Sure'.

Then he kept driving, saying that he wanted to show me something else. We stopped at a lodge with a view of the coastline.

He pointed at the view and said, 'Wouldn't you just love seeing the sunsets here every night?'

I said, 'Sure'.

He took me to a few different places, each time asking how great it would be to do this and that there. He drove us right up to the beach and I stopped him before he could finish telling me that he had something to show me.

'What are we doing?', I asked, getting annoyed.

He spontaneously said, 'Let's go swimming!'

He was clearly avoiding talking about something that he was building up to with his various detours.

It was freezing, so I replied, 'Hell no! What do you have to show me? Just tell me.'

Aaron started walking towards the ocean and when he noticed I hadn't followed behind, he ran back to me. It was too cold for the water but the beach was still beautiful. As we stood together, he told me how much he loved me and then got down onto one knee before pulling out a paperclip wrapped into a ring. When we started dating, I never wore my seatbelt and when he told me to put it on, I would point to my bare ring finger, twist my hand back and forth, and say he couldn't tell me what to do yet. One time, he got so annoyed that he pulled out a paperclip, made it into a ring, and shoved it on my finger. I had no comeback to that, so I started wearing my seatbelt.

He said there was a real ring for me, but he thought the paperclip ring was much more special at that moment. I was ecstatic and immediately said yes. I would have happily walked around with the paperclip on for months, but the real ring was beautiful. It has our birthstones, his parents', my mom's, and Steve's, and our two names engraved on the side. So, I had two paperclip rings (I kept the original), a meaningful engagement ring, and a husband-to-be.

We chose a date that night and sent out our save the dates the next day. My apartment lease was up in July, so we decided to get married and move in together before then.

Aaron told our families that he was planning to propose two months earlier, and both of our moms were upset that there were no photos of the proposal. Neither of us wanted that because we valued the intimacy of our precious moment. We had engagement photos taken on April 6th by our friend Alesha. She's so sweet and a good friend to Aaron and I. We had so much fun doing that photoshoot and we took fake proposal photos to make our moms happy.

On April 15th, I picked my dress. Two weeks before Aaron proposed, I had been scrolling through wedding dresses for fun and had saved my favorite idea. When I went into the wedding dress store, I showed them that photo and found my dream dress. The bodice was made up of cascading white leaves, lined with diamantes, that flowed down into a big tulle skirt with peachy undertones. My mom, mother-in-law Gail, Emilie, and maid of honor Kaylee all loved it but of course, Olivia who was on Facetime wasn't a fan. Emilie and Kaylee picked the bridesmaid's dresses and Emilie's choices were a little too teenaged or busty for the other bridesmaids. They settled on silky maxi dresses in the gorgeous dusky shade of red that our color scheme became based on.

I got my bridal party some gifts to say thank you. Gail adores turquoise so I got her a turquoise necklace with earrings and my mom got a ruby necklace with a stone for each of her children. I remember getting Emilie a little hand-crafted hunting knife because she loves unique things like that.

On April 22nd, my women's bible study group threw me a bachelorette party. It was hilariously fun and very clean, although I did get some mild lingerie, as is a rite of passage for a bride-to-be. My mom, Gail, and Kaylee threw me a bridal shower at our wedding venue, Shady Oaks. The venue is owned by Kaylee's grandparents, and it was where we had Mother's Day lunch back in 2019. For the bridal shower, one of my friends made a chocolate heart with silhouettes of a bride and groom standing under an intricate arch. It was one that you crack open to get the gift inside, but they had to force me to break it because it was just too pretty.

The rehearsal dinner was the day before the wedding. Our venue has a little fairytale-style bridge and Aaron decided he wanted to walk everyone over that bridge to their seats. Jamie (our good friend and venue decorator) noticed I could come in from the back, hidden at first by the trees, and make a grand entrance surrounded by beautiful blooming flowers. So, I kept that in my back pocket to surprise Aaron.

Our wedding day was June 26th, 2021. Olivia did my and the other bridesmaid's hair and makeup as her gift because she's a professional makeup artist and hairdresser. My hair is naturally curly and usually bunches up into big curly locks. But in 109°F weather, my hair decided that for the first time, it wanted to be incredibly straight and flat. Olivia spent ages trying to get it curled but no amount of hairspray made them stick. The most frustrating part was that I woke up with gorgeous curls the next day.

My mom helped us girls get ready, and she was a godsend when Kaylee's bridesmaid dress ripped that morning. Mom got me into my dress and then she and Olivia put my necklace on together.

When I was ready, she looked at me with such love in her eyes and said, 'When you get to the end of that aisle, you tell Aaron that I said you were right.'

I laughed, kissed her, and knew that this woman raised me to be a good woman and future wife.

Despite it being rock hard with hairspray and holding no curls, my hair flowed down my back in waves with a glistening tiara on top. It was a gloriously sunny day and the summer sun lit up each diamante on my tiara and dress. I felt like a princess and because I grew up unsure if I would get to have a wedding, that was the most special feeling. That entire day just felt like a dream. I couldn't believe I had made it and that I would get to marry my best friend.

As I walked towards the aisle, I remember Aaron looking towards the bridge for me with a little disappointment because he couldn't see me anywhere. As soon as he saw me emerge from the trees, his eyes poured like waterfalls, and he was trying to stop but his face just contorted in the funniest ways. I started crying too, with my men in black beside me. My dad and stepdad both walked me down the aisle in black suits with almost matching black sunglasses, and they looked like my security detail.

Everything had been simple and easy because we had so much help from family and friends. We just wanted a small celebration with us and God, but everyone else made it even more special. Our friend was the DJ, my mom's friend made the cakes, our friend Jamie set up the decorations, a kind lady from church put together all of our flowers and our good friend who's a pastor officiated.

There were so many precious moments during our wedding day.

For the three months of our engagement, I tried teaching Zan, the girl I took care of, how to throw flowers because she was our flower girl. We would pretend that the hallway was the aisle but instead of sprinkling the petals around, she would either refuse or dump them all on the ground. That didn't actually matter to me, I just wanted her to be part of our wedding. However, that day, I watched from behind the bushes as she stopped and turned to face the guests before sprinkling petals at each row. She did it the whole way down until her sister, and my bridesmaid, Kaylee, helped her to her seat. It was the most beautiful thing. I was so proud of her.

Zan walked down the aisle alongside Zi, our ring bearer and family friend who had a huge crush on me. As they walked back down the aisle, Zan had the biggest smile and was so excited to get to do it all over again. Whereas, Zi had the biggest pout because he was miserable after having just watched me marry someone other than him.

The wedding ring that Zi carried was the plain wedding band that I had chosen. I had always wished to eventually use my Nana's wedding ring which was from Ukraine. I wanted it for my wedding because I was the grandchild that Nana was closest to and it meant a lot to me. However, it had been passed down to Jacob after Aunt Tammy passed. I often told Jacob that I loved that ring, especially while I was wedding planning, but he wanted to keep it, so I bought a new one. At the rehearsal dinner, Jacob showed up with that ring in his pocket and gave it to Aaron. On our wedding day, Aaron surprised me with it after Zi passed us the plain ring. So, I got my Nana's special ring after all. Aaron has an equally meaningful ring because it has blue and green inside of it- the IIH colors.

I don't remember much of our vows, but one part of Aaron's vows that I will never forget is his tribute to how many times I have escaped death.

He joked that I stared death down with a shotgun many times throughout our relationship and every time said, 'Nope, not today.'

That's something I plan to keep on doing for as long as I can. Our ceremony was an unforgettable moment in which we both had nothing but pure appreciation, love, and good jokes for each other.

The day before the wedding, I said to Aaron, 'Let's be cool and different.'

He laughed, 'I'm marrying someone who's had countless brain surgeries, how can I be more different than that?'

I said, 'No, I mean let's skip down the aisle!'

After the ceremony, we did. We intertwined our hands and skipped down the aisle like a couple of kids. My mom's face screwed up into a ball of irritation because she wanted us to do it properly and get pretty photos taken. However, Alesha captured my dress floating in the wind as we skipped away, and that photo is now proudly displayed all over my mom's house. It ended up becoming her favorite photo.

After that, we had lots of family photos taken, had some food and then we had our first dance before speeches.

Our song was Aerosmith's 'I Don't Want to Miss a Thing' because when we were dating, we used to listen to that song and after Aaron realized how ill I was, he would say that he really didn't want to miss a thing. We had a beautiful first dance to that song. Then I danced individually with my dad, Steve, and my father-in-law Chuck too. Aaron, on the other hand, danced with my mom, his mom, and Emilie.

When the time came to cut the cake, we couldn't. We tried pushing the knife in so hard, but it just wouldn't cut. We were laughing and beginning to think that the cake had been replaced with bricks. Once we figured out that we were trying to cut the plastic board between the layers, we got it. Aaron had said in advance that he didn't want to do the tacky tradition of smashing wedding cake into each other's faces, and we agreed on that. But when the time came, I wasn't sure if he had said that to throw me off the scent and we stood there with our pieces of cake, both laughing with a hint of anxiety. Eventually, I trusted him enough to take a bite and then I started eating my own piece, so he had to remind me that we're supposed to keep feeding each other. We didn't do too well with the cake traditions.

We had a dry wedding without a huge party because a few of our guests were alcoholics and many were older people with no interest in alcohol. Plus we just wanted a calm wedding. So, we had a sunny reception with lots of food, chatting and speeches.

My bridesmaid Kaylee gave a lovely speech that I still have folded up in my jewelry box. Emilie gave a gorgeous little speech and then came Olivia's. She started by saying that she had written a speech on the flight because if the younger sister was getting married first, she had to write a speech for it.

It was surprisingly sweet and right at the end, she said, 'Aaron, after all these years, you can finally hug me.'

He immediately shot out of his seat and enclosed her in the biggest hug until she shooed him off. That was so special because it was like she officially accepted him as her brother-in-law.

While everyone was mingling, my little step-niece Mia ran up to me and asked what I was eating, and I replied, 'A cupcake, you want some?'

I shoved it right in her face and her giggle was adorable. I mean it was a wedding, so somebody had to get cake in their face.

Our photographer Alesha snapped the perfect photo of her laughing with white icing smeared all over her face before Mia shouted, 'Auntie Jackie, look what the bride did!'.

That night, we were like a couple of kids on Christmas morning. We sat and opened every single present until our hotel room was trashed with wrapping paper and boxes. One gift I remember is that Dr. Knives got us a fancy block of knives. Of course, that's not his real name but knives were still an ironic gift to get from your neurosurgeon. Barry from Denver Children's Hospital all those years ago also got us a gift. It was lovely to see just how many people thought of us on our big day. That big day was more perfect than I ever could have imagined, and I will always cherish it more than anything.

Chapter Ten

A fter four years of growing our bond, making countless memories, and holding each other's hands through the toughest of times, we were officially husband and wife. Our honeymoon wasn't planned until months later because my health, work, and Aaron's work didn't allow for such a short notice trip. Instead, Aaron's boss had paid for us to go to an expensive restaurant in Bend.

On July 7th, we drove to Downtown Bend for the evening. I wore my little white wedding after-party dress and Aaron wore a nice suit. After the fancy meal for which Aaron's boss had kindly spared no expense, we walked through the town. We came across a group of younger girls who complimented our outfits and offered to take a photo of us. We watched as they spent about ten minutes contorting themselves all over the room to get the perfect angles and leave us with twenty photos. It's safe to say that those fabulous girls belonged to the social media era.

It was a thirty-minute drive home and I had to use the bathroom before we were five minutes into the journey. The only place nearby was Planet Fitness, so I walked in wearing an elegant white dress and strolled past a gym full of sweaty people judging me. That membership came in handy.

My 23r^d birthday was a week later on July 14th and Jacob came to visit. Aaron was working, so Jacob and I had the whole afternoon to fill. First of all, Jacob is Mercury's original dad, so he was really coming to see her. They spent some time together and we tried to get a photo with all of us, but we just got a photo of us trying to catch her as she leaped away mid-air. We went out to breakfast in Sunriver before visiting a mountain peak which enveloped us in trees and then we discovered a nearby restaurant which sat on a beautiful lake. We had lunch basking under the sun's warmth and watching the water ripple under its orange glow. Afterward, we went to waste time joking around at Walmart until Aaron got home and then we competed playing video games all night. Life had felt unusually peaceful since the last surgery and while I knew it would be short-lived, I was making the most of it.

On July 20th, I flew to Ohio to surprise my Nana Nadia (My Nana's sister). I had four days off work and realized how long it had been since I last visited her, so I did just that. She was so excited to find me on the other side of her door. While I was there, I got to meet someone else who meant a lot to me. When I first got diagnosed, I made friends online with another teenager with IIH who lived in Ohio. Although the condition had blinded him, he could type by feeling the keys and we would talk all the time. We didn't get to be friends for very long. I remember when he passed, Aaron wrote me a condolence card even though we hadn't become friends yet. I also knew Evan's mom, Ruth, and she was my pen pal even after Evan passed away. They both taught me a lot about IIH and while I was sad to have never met Evan, meeting Ruth was precious.

I filled that summer with so many memories. When we lived in Wyoming, my family would visit Yellowstone regularly, and as a teenager, I complained that it was boring and smelt of rotten eggs but by 23 years old, I missed it. So, we found the next best thing- the deepest lake in the USA. We drove an hour and a half to visit the volcanic Crater Lake in Oregon. However, the wildfires meant that it was hidden beneath a thick fog, and we didn't see a thing. To make up for that, we visited the Big Obsidian Flow, which is a lava flow. The obsidian stones on top of the mountain looked magical. I walked down the steep mountainside to sit on the edge and be enveloped in the open air and greenery for a moment. Despite Aaron's very loud anxiety, I did not fall off the mountain. There were signs asking people not to take the rocks, but I always take a little token from wherever I visit, and this one felt special, so I asked Aaron if I could take one. He said no because if people saw it could start a chain reaction. It would take so many people to make that unlikely chain reaction noticeable, but I said fine.

When we got back in the car, I turned to Aaron with a little shiny black thing and said, 'Look at my little rock!'

He told me off, but I just said he could take it back when I'm gone. I agree that you shouldn't take things when you're asked not to, but I think there should be some leeway for a terminally ill person who intends to have it returned with no harm done. After the Big Obsidian Flow, Aaron took me to try his virtual reality headset for the first time. He put it on me, made me play a plank game, and started recording. I hesitantly shuffled along this virtual board to reach a cake and when I got there, Aaron told me to take a bite. As I did, a huge spider jumped out onto my face and I frantically shuffled backward as Aaron stood there thinking *wow, this was a great idea*.

At the end of August, Emilie spent a weekend with us. First, took her to an obstacle course. While Emilie and Aaron sped through the hurdles, I kept letting everyone go ahead of me until I had to go because they were waiting for me. That probably wasn't the best activity with two shunts, but it was exhaustingly fun. Then, we visited a zoo where Emilie and I adopted an otter for a year because we were obsessed with how adorable they were. That was the last of our 2021 adventures in Oregon, before Aaron and I moved to Donna, Texas.

Aaron's job at the time was in RV sales and during the colder months in Bend, there was very little desire for RVs. However, there is a market for RVs in Texas during the winter, so in October, we packed up and moved. Our three cats came with us, two traveled in cat carriers while Mercury the car cat enjoyed the journey from my lap. I loved living in Donna. While Aaron worked in the office, he could see me sunbathing through the window and would text me, 'By the pool again, huh?' We ended up living there for three months and I spent almost every day by the pool in a relaxing 55 and up park. I made friends with this delightful old lady who was so tanned and wrinkled that she reminded me of a lovely little raisin. We went to craft fairs and hung out by the pool together. It was bliss... well, maybe not for Aaron who was stuck in the office.

I was scheduled to have surgery back home in Oregon at the beginning of December. It was a simple little surgery compared to the others. The Chiari surgery hadn't worked properly. My brain was still falling, partially because my LP shunt was pulling out so much CSF that it was pulling my brain down with it. The plan was to go into my LP shunt and clamp it- simple enough and no need for Aaron to miss work to accompany me. However, when I flew down to Eugene on December 9th, I got one false positive COVID test and they had to cancel the surgery for at least 30 days. Due to COVID restrictions, I wasn't allowed to fly back to Aaron for 14 days, so I stayed at my mom's house in Eugene. During that time, his job relocated him again, so he was busy transferring to Arizona. So, we had to spend our first Christmas as a married couple apart. My family did our usual Christmas traditions, and it was lovely, but I missed Aaron. On December 31st, I finally flew to Arizona to see Aaron in Cottonwood. I stayed with him until January 9th and then I had to fly back to Eugene for the simple surgery.

This time when I got to Eugene, I stayed with my in-laws so that I could spend some time with them. Aaron's dad Chuck is such a good soul that he goes woodcutting to provide firewood for families in need, and I remember him doing that while I stayed there. I also remember that he asked me to help him take down the Christmas lights.

He asked me to reel up this long orange extension cord, so I started winding it up and he yelled down from the ladder, 'What are you doing?'

He told me that I was doing it wrong and had to unreel it and then stretch it out across the yard before reeling it up again. I asked what the difference was but apparently, that was just the 'right' way.

I replied, 'Okay, Dad. Next time, I'm not helping if I just do it wrong.'

After that, he took me into his shop to show off how nice it looked.

I was like, 'But what are all these boxes?'

He said it was all important stuff, but he was just hoarding it. I joked about it every day until he finally started clearing everything out. Aaron's mom, Gail, is convinced that I have some kind of magic touch with Chuck because she could never get him to get rid of stuff. He still texts me pictures of his decluttering to prove that he's doing it. Chuck's quirkiness is brilliant; he's such a lovable kooky guy and Gail is like a second mom to me. I missed Aaron again, but spending time with his family made me feel better.

On January 18th, 2022, my mom took me for the surgery. They went into my spine and clamped the shunt off. The easy surgery was accomplished. That night, my mom and I stayed at a nearby hotel. I told my mom that my eyes were hurting, and I felt nauseous. It got worse until I couldn't open my eyes, talk, or comprehend much of anything. My mom called an ambulance and got the paramedics sent to our room. I don't remember any of that night, but I'm told that there were four paramedics. They asked if I could move, but I couldn't. My mom explained the situation to them, and they immediately got me into the ambulance. She called Aaron and said he needed to get there, which was frustrating because it was a simple surgery, so he hadn't arranged time off work. Despite that fact, he turned up at the hospital the next day.

Dr. D discovered that my brain had moved back into its designated spot within 18 hours. That amount of movement should have taken days or even weeks. He didn't know what to do because that never should have happened and my pressure was far too high. However, if he just unclamped the shunt, my brain could have been pulled back down dangerously fast. So, I spent a lot of time in the hospital getting spinal taps to relieve the pressure while they figured out what to do. By the end of that ordeal, they had to start going three spots lower than the original spinal tap region because the tissue had been gradually destroyed by my 300-plus spinal taps. I left the hospital on January 30th under the agreement that I would keep coming back for spinal taps until the next surgery slot on February 9th. Shunts were not made for my illness and valves were not made for LP shunts, so it was like sticking tape over a burst pipe and hoping it would hold. Unsurprisingly, they found that my valve had broken. Determined to persevere the shunt, they replaced the valve again. This time, Dr. D used a bubble mechanism valve. It had little bubbles in it that would help regulate my pressure by making the CSF flow more when I sat up and less when I lay down. So, I was fixed up again for a little while.

I got out of the hospital on February 10th and stayed with my in-laws again for a few days. Aaron flew out for our first married Valentine's Day but then he had to fly straight back to Arizona. I migrated to my mom's house so that I could spend more time with my family too. On my last day in Eugene, I took my niece Mia out for the day. We went to a fair where I bought her homemade playdough that smelled like strawberries and cupcakes, we got a caricature done, and then I took her to dinner. The whole day people mistook us for mother and daughter because we look so alike. After a while, I got tired of correcting them, so I told her to just go with it and I had a kid for the day. I loved that day, but what I loved most was flying to Arizona to be with Aaron and our kitties. With a small break from surgeries, Aaron and I got to explore Arizona together and our honeymoon was finally just around the corner. It was time to enjoy life again.

Chapter Eleven

O
ur adventures began in Prescott where we visited The Palace, an old-fashioned saloon with some of the best beer around. Next was Sedona where we saw all the local attractions including the Pueblos. My favorite was the Wupatki National Monument because you could stand in the dusty ruins where a community thrived thousands of years ago. On March 15th, we stayed on an Indian reservation near Horseshoe Bend, Arizona. For two nights, we slept in a wagon with no electricity or bathroom. There were mud huts, teepees, tents, and wagons. We thought the reliance on nature would be cool, but I was not a fan of the bucket of water that was left to warm up in the sun for everybody to share for showers. Needless to say, I didn't shower while we were there. At night, it was so cold and pitch black, but in the mornings, the hosts made us the most amazing breakfasts. They made the coffee themselves and cooked the food over a firepit. While we stayed there, we visited Horseshoe Bend, the Grand Canyon, and the Antelope Canyon which we were lucky to get a last-minute slot for. The Antelope Canyon was beautiful and part of the natural stone was shaped like a lion and one part like an upside-down heart. We weren't allowed to take many photographs due to it being native land, but I could never forget those sights. Our final Arizona adventure was Jerome. We took a motorcycle and it was freeing to drift through the

wind on those empty, winding roads. We visited Gold King Mine & Ghost Town which was interesting because they had the old equipment used to pull teeth or sew. Other than that, it was essentially a junkyard, which made it feel more like a ghost town. I loved exploring Arizona with Aaron but I unwillingly took a break back to reality.

I had to travel from Cottonwood, Arizona, back to Bend, Oregon on March 26th in time for another appointment. It was such a long journey and I had the cats with me too, so I had to stop at a hotel en route in Round Mountain. It was the kind of hotel that looked like a horror movie set. When I got to Bend, I stayed at a much more comfortable little cabin. The next day, I had an MRI scan for a lump on my back that looked suspiciously like a CSF leak. It was. They decided to give me an awful corset in an attempt to push the CSF leak back in. They thought the fluid could be coming out and around the shunt rather than going into it. So, I begrudgingly took the corset and had to wear it as much as I could bear in the insanely hot spring weather. I also had to wear it over a shirt rather than under, so It wasn't very subtle.

On April 1st, my cousin Nicole provided a needed distraction by visiting for a couple of days. We spent the whole time making girly trips: shopping, getting yogurt, and seeing all the tourist spots that I knew of. My part in the shopping was getting outfits for the honeymoon which was in just a few weeks. On April 12th, Aaron finally moved back home and he brought three inches of snow with him which was somehow right in the middle of a spring heatwave. The weird weather helped me keep that corset on though because it had been too warm to wear it. That day, we also got the offer of our third cat, Spunky. Aaron had been asking for another cat for ages but I wasn't convinced. Then, we get photos of adorable kittens asking us to be their parents- I mean come on! I agreed to think about it, which kept Aaron happy. On Easter Sunday, we went to church with our RV friends the Mclaughlins. Aaron wore a nice suit and I got dressed up but refused to wear the corset too. On the 21st, the kittens' owner brought them to Aaron's work and told us to pick one. I picked the cute little one that she held in her hand, but she said I couldn't have that one.

I was like, 'Oh, okay, so I can't pick.'

I went for the little white one with some colorful patches, but she didn't like to be held and ended up running around the place causing mayhem. That little nightmare ended up being ours.

On April 30th, our honeymoon finally arrived and we were so excited to spend just over two weeks in Cancun together. I took the corset with me and Aaron kept telling me to wear it, but it was so hot that I would have melted if I wore it. Aaron slept on the flight as usual and when we got off the plane, everything was so bright, warm, and blue. Our balcony overlooked the pool, the forestry, and the ocean. We enjoyed sitting there and people-watching, outfit judging, watching the evening shows, and taking in the view. However, they had pool parties that ran until 5 am and we learned how truly old we are because we complained like a wrinkled-up couple when we couldn't get our peaceful 10 pm bedtime. The pool did have its good qualities, for example, there was a swim-up bar where we learned that if you tip your bartender well, your drinks come extra strong and make the day even more fun. At the start of our stay, we went to some timeshare spiel that gave us an amazing free lunch and magnificent views of the ocean. It was well worth the hour of sales pitches which we had no intention of actually partaking in.

Our first day trip was to Chichén Itzá, which I can never remember the pronunciation of so I say, 'Hey, Aaron, remember that time we went to Chicken Pizza?'

When you stood at the end of the ruins and clapped, it sounded like a bird. It was hilarious that there were a bunch of people clapping at the building followed by a bombardment of chirps. We also visited a Mexican restaurant where ladies do an authentic Mexican dance with bottles balanced on their heads. I was in awe because there was a 0% chance that those would remain intact if I tried. Then, we visited a Yucatan Cenote which was a natural sinkhole and sacred water source for the Mayans. We entered halfway into the hole and it went miles up to the open blue sky and ages down to a waterfall and a circular pool. I couldn't convince Aaron to go swimming with me, so I explored the freezing water by myself. It was such a serene moment to stand under the waterfall and feel the cool water on my skin while hearing the splashes echo miles above me. Whenever I climb the steps out of a pool of any sort, Aaron loves to take a photo of me, and he followed tradition that time.

He showed it to me, smirking proudly, and said, 'Doesn't your butt look great in this?'

'Where am I?', I asked.

He pointed to a girl in a red bikini. I stared at him and slowly asked, 'What color is my swimsuit, Aaron?'

He examined me, then the photo, then me again, and with wide eyes he said, 'You're wearing blue.'

He's the perfect doting husband, just to the wrong woman that time. It was hilarious and I still love to remind him of it.

After that trip, we went to another timeshare to see what free stuff we could get. They agreed that if we listened to their spiel for one hour, we would get free tickets to a nearby adventure park called Xplor. We sat through one hour, but they refused to give us the tickets, so Aaron wandered off and I stayed to bicker until they eventually gave me the tickets and showed us to the park. We went on five different ziplines through the forestry, went on a huge waterslide, and raced ATVs around the park. They kept telling us to slow down but we were having too much fun. When I was driving, one of the cameras snapped a photo of Aaron screaming while grabbing onto the railing for his life. At one point, we had to go through a cave with a group of people to get to the next destination. When we were walking, the glowing blue water came pretty high up on me compared to the tall people. We also had to use a hand-paddled raft through the cave, and we kept bumping into people because we couldn't paddle the thing in the right direction at the same time. Xplor was so cool and well worth the hour of timeshare talk.

On a ridiculously hot day, we took a dollar bus ride to a beachfront zoo and saw a bunch of flamingos, parrots, hatching baby quails, lemurs, and string rays. The next day, we took a boat ride to Isla Mujeres, a little nearby town that had the most amazing one-dollar tacos. Every evening, we had dinner at sunset and got dressed up. I remember struggling to tame my hair when we dressed up because the humidity made it uncontrollably frizzy.

One day during our honeymoon, we went to go and do something that I had always dreamed of. We went to Quintana Roo to swim with dolphins. I had missed out on that experience in Las Vegas in 2015 and I finally got to make up for that. First, they kissed me, then pulled me across the water with their dorsal fins, and then we got to stroke their flippers before doing a pose with them. We both chose Superman, but Aaron's looked more convincing. The final trick that they did was letting us put our feet on their noses so they could lift us into the air. Aaron got it the first time, but you have to relax your whole body and trust that you won't fall or drown and I couldn't manage that. I kept trying but it was also physically difficult and on the fourth time, they said it would have to be my final attempt. Thankfully, I got it and now we have a photo of me sailing above the water with an expression of utter joy.

The final excursion of our honeymoon was parasailing. Aaron wanted to go scuba diving, but I couldn't do that due to the pressure changes in deep water, so we agreed on parasailing instead. (Sadly, there are things I can't do because of IIH. Sometimes I don't do those things... other times I do). We had this huge yellow parasail with a big blue smiley face on it and Aaron's legs dangled down all relaxed as mine curled up in a tense ball. It was cool though, we got to see so much of Cancun's coastline up there.

On May 14th, we came home feeling fulfilled and rested. The perfect time to introduce a feisty new kitten to the house. Not only was our relaxation interrupted by Spunky, but I only had a couple of days at home before traveling to Washington DC with Emilie as her school trip chaperone. However, we had a great time on that school trip together. The bus took us everywhere including New York and Maryland. One day, we were on the bus until 3 am and I would have been happy to call it a day and sleep there, but we arrived at a hotel without enough rooms. I wanted to get to bed so I agreed to take a couple of extra kids but they took so long to decide who that I rescinded my offer, took the key and Emilie, and slunk off to bed. I was under the impression that with a 3 am bedtime, we would be able to sleep until maybe 9 am. Nope, they allowed us three hours of sleep.

On the honeymoon, I was starting to hurt pretty bad but this trip was completely non-stop. The lump on my back was starting to go away, but there was a new, small lump on my side that was very painful and I was taking photos of it every day to monitor the growth. There was one opportunity for me to have a day at the hotel, so I got someone else to chaperone Emilie, rested in bed all day, and met up for dinner later. Regardless of the exhaustion and pain that I was in, I never regretted taking Emilie on that trip because we had the most precious one-on-one bonding time. Every night, we would get into bed and record everything we did so that I could never forget. I don't remember everything, so I'm glad that it's all there for us to relive together.

I got back to Bend, Oregon on June 4th, and after a long trip away from Aaron, it was nice to be home. Our first wedding Anniversary was soon after. We get anniversary photos every year so that we can see ourselves grow and if I manage to survive until we're old and grey, we can look back on our life together. The reality is that it will likely just be Aaron looking back on us, but he will have lots of photos to keep those memories alive. After our photoshoot, we went away to a farm in Eugene which had a gorgeous rustic barn, a tree swing, and animals. It was my mom and stepdad's gift to us and it was lovely; we couldn't have been more thankful. The sweet host made us a 'Happy Anniversary' cake and presented it alongside champagne and a cheese board. There had been two swans on the farm's lake and they were mated for life, so after one had died, the other remained alone. He made for good company though. We loved it there and we're planning to hold our fifth-anniversary vow renewal there. Normally people renew their vows on their tenth anniversary, but I probably won't make it until then so we settled on halfway. I couldn't believe that we had been husband and wife for an entire year, and what a year it had been.

Chapter Twelve

The summer of 2022 brought my 24th birthday and Aaron gave me a tennis bracelet with 40 tiny sparkling diamonds, one for each of my surgeries. While we wanted a quiet celebration, life had other plans. In Oregon, you never hang out in the rivers because you can freeze or easily get caught in the currents. A few young girls had gone to play in the lake away from their parents and had gotten lost. We helped the police in their search because Aaron had a drone. We flew it over a wide span of the river and eventually saw them waving for help. There was no way to communicate, so we hovered the drone above them and used it to lead them to a safe place to get out with less risk of drowning. We ended up in the newspaper for that, but it was the least we could do to help those girls.

A few days after my birthday, I had an LFT CTR and MP decompression, which is treatment for Myalgia Prosthetica and carpel tunnel. The carpel tunnel surgery was fine, but they had to go in and cut the nerve at the top of my leg meaning I couldn't walk for two weeks. Compared to the other surgeries it was nothing, but it sucked to be stuck on the sofa unable to do anything but read. I read a *lot*. My leg is still pretty bad so I have to decide if I want them to go back in and cut the nerve completely. Although, I could end up with no feeling in my leg and I think I would rather have pain than nothing at all.

Once I was healed, we started building Aaron's birthday present at the end of August. His birthday is in November, but he would not stop talking about wanting to brew beer like he used to, so I gave in and we started building. There was a study space in our trailer that we never really used, so we ripped it out, built walls, and re-did the floor with dark-stained wood. We used a freezer as the base for the bottles and kegs and put the keezer next to it. It rotates so that we can pour the beer out of the back window when we're outside. Funnily enough, we don't drink beer. Aaron just enjoys brewing it, so we gift it to everybody. Dr. D liked it so much that he asked for more. Alcohol is the typical gift for your neurosurgeon, right?

We were due to move to Mount Hood in early October, so when Boy Kitty ran away right before that, it wasn't ideal. He had been trying to get to a squirrel and as soon as the door opened a crack, he saw his opportunity and bolted. Late September was getting cold and moving day was getting close so we had to find him. At first, we called him and left out a trap with food in it but instead, we caught a bunny. On day five, we went outside to call him and shake treats. As I walked around calling him, I could hear him meowing, but Aaron insisted there was no noise. I sat down feeling defeated. Aaron suddenly said that he heard it, so we got back up and started frantically looking for him. We figured out that he had climbed through the hole in the bottom of the RV to get back inside, but got stuck in the belly of the RV. Aaron had to rip apart the floor to get him out. After that, our freezing little Boy Kitty laid on a heating pad for hours and became terrified of everything.

On October 11th, we moved to Mount Hood for Aaron's job. We were closer to my doctors, but further away from our friends and family. Despite being away from everything, we made Halloween as fun as always. Every year, we make a big deal of Halloween to celebrate the anniversary of my first shunt surgery. That year, we went all out and dressed up as Sandy and Danny from Grease.

Winter was fast approaching and over the last couple of months, I had pretty much forgotten about that corset brace that I was supposed to be wearing. I had worn it for a considerable amount of time, especially while on Emilie's school trip. The summer heat had been difficult enough without it and by the autumn, I just wanted to live life without the added hassle. Unsurprisingly, my lump had gotten big enough for my mom to start calling it my camel hump. Three days after Aaron's birthday on November 8th, I had surgery to fix it. In the surgery room, they usually ask you what you're having done, and what your allergies are, and then they put you to sleep. With me, they also chitchat for a while and my anaesthesiologist even sings to me to put me to sleep. (One sang to me in 2019 and now I insist they all do it. When I ask them, they usually make me repeat the request out of disbelief). They were in the middle of putting me to sleep and someone suddenly shouted stop. They took my oxygen mask off and a lady started asking me about my interests. I ignored her questions and asked what was going on. She said Dr. D needed to talk to me first.

Then I said, 'Okay, now we can chit-chat.'

We chatted for a while until Dr. D arrived and apologized. He said that seeing as I hadn't had much luck with the bubble mechanism valve, they had designed a magnetically adjustable valve just for me. He gave me the choice of replacing the current bubble mechanism valve or trying the new valve. We decided on the new one and I was finally put to sleep. I woke up to learn that the leak had been caused by my LP catheter tubing being out by just 1mm. Fortunately, I only lost two days to the hospital for that visit. Although, ten days later, they had to adjust the valve due to high-pressure headaches.

My family booked a holiday to stay near us in Mount Hood for Thanksgiving. On Thanksgiving morning, we were going to go on a train ride and then pottery painting. Everyone was getting ready. Emilie and Aaron were nearby in the kitchen while I was sitting next to Zac on the couch, eating a small pastry-like cake. All of a sudden, I realized I couldn't breathe. The cake lodged itself in my throat as I tried to gasp for air. Zac didn't know what to do and Emilie screamed for Mom and Steve. I started turning blue. Aaron did the Heimlich maneuver and saved my life, then he sat me down and asked if I was okay. I was not okay; I was in a lot of pain and my ribs were badly bruised. I said I was fine and just needed a breather before going out. Also, I did not finish that cake. I couldn't believe that after countless brain surgeries, a cake almost took me out. Anyway, we went on the train ride and met people from Bend. Aaron told them that he saved my life and probably broke my ribs and they looked at me thinking, *Why are you here right now?* I reassured them I was fine, through gritted teeth, while hunched over. So, we continued on to pottery painting and assumed everything was fine.

On December 6th, I noticed a little lump on my side where my LP shunt valve is. It was tiny, so I took a photo for monitoring and moved on. On the 18th, I realized that the lump had gotten much bigger. I called my doctor and he ordered a CT scan, which took a few weeks to go through insurance and get scheduled. While we waited, Christmas provided a much-needed distraction. We went to my parents' house for Christmas Eve and joined Aaron's parents for Christmas Day. At my mom's house, we did our usual Secret Santa and a bingo game where the winner gets a stocking with a gift card in it. Christmas at Aaron's parent's house was much more relaxed. They don't usually buy gifts, but they know that gift-giving is my love language, so I always get one. We followed their tradition of eating prime rib and watched the same soppy movie that Gail chooses every year. Aaron and I have our own tradition, which is to go and look at all the rich people's ridiculously fabulous Christmas lights because I adore them. A few days after Christmas, we noticed that my lump was getting even bigger. It was huge at this point and I couldn't lay on my side, touch my side, or wear clothes that touched it. I hid beneath big sweaters to disguise it.

Despite that pain, Aaron and I started 2023 with a weekend away in a beautiful hotel where each room had a unique name and old wooden beams with antique fireplaces. After that, Gail and I went on a six-and-a-half-hour drive to visit Aaron's aunt Carolyn.

On the journey, we passed windmills and Gail said, 'Look at the baby ones!' and we laughed.

When Aaron and I moved to Texas his parents came with us and I said, 'Aww look at the baby windmills!'

Gail had replied, 'They're not babies, they're just far away.'

Then she realized that they were tiny windmills and now we joke whenever we see windmills.

After seeing Aunt Carolyn, Gail and I stayed in a hotel and had girly chats for hours. It was a lovely little trip.

Reality resumed on February 7th, when I had surgery to fix the second lump. The doctors had to do a nuclear med study, where they put dye into my IV and then scan me to see what's happening in there. It showed that CSF was free-flowing into my side because my LP shunt was broken. When Aaron did the Heimlich maneuver, he managed to rotate my valve in a full circle so that it broke and the catheter got pulled out. The med study made it look like the catheter tubing was still attached, but when they opened me up, it wasn't. During that surgery, they had to dig into my side to create a pocket of flesh for my valve to sit in to avoid future damage. That part was particularly painful to recover from. Since then, I haven't had any huge leaks. That leak was bigger than a golf ball, so I can understand why they had to protect the valve. The doctors didn't blame Aaron entirely, but it was quite obvious that his saving my life caused it. I'm very glad that he did, but it's safe to say that I never want a repeat of that whole thing again.

That surgery left me in the hospital until February 15th. What I hated the most was that Dr. D had to make a six-inch incision down my Nana's memorial tattoo. I've had that tattoo since I was 15 years old, and even though it was very painful, I chose the placement on my ribs because I thought it would never get cut into. I couldn't say no when Dr. D asked but I was devastated to see it cut into. However, Dr. D kindly did a particularly neat job. I hadn't had any time off before that surgery and my boss didn't know until then that anything was wrong. I had just been extra careful when looking after the child to make sure nothing touched my side. I couldn't stick a smile on and go to work for a little while after that surgery.

For the rest of our time living in Mount Hood, we led boring yet hectic lives. Work, doctor's appointments, work on the rental house, collapse on the sofa, sleep, repeat. We hated it. The location was lovely, but we had no time to ourselves and even if we did, it wasn't easy to just pop to a friend's house when we lived so far away.

My job is to take care of a disabled little girl on weekends to give her parents some respite. I would usually leave for work on Thursdays at 7 pm, but living in Mount Hood, I had to leave at 11 am to get there before it was completely dark. That's part of the reason that living in Bend is perfect for us. While I find my job very physically taxing, it's great to see her parents have the freedom to go fishing (even with multiple freezers full of fish), join quilting classes, or spend time with their four young grandchildren. They're very accommodating with my health too, so it's pretty much the perfect part-time job for me.

At the end of February, Aaron found time to go to a couple of RV shows in Seattle and I went with him, but I spent most of my time in the hotel room. I was still recovering, but we did get to go for a lovely dinner together while we were there. I hadn't had my stitches pulled out yet and while it might have been more uncomfortable to have the stitches in, I wasn't looking forward to the removal process.

After that tiny trip, we arrived home to a call from the tenants of our rental house telling us that the heating was broken. So we had to drive to Eugene at 3 am, in the middle of a snowstorm. We tried to get the main fireplace working and had to go out to get space heaters for each tenant's room. That was just what I needed mid-recovery.

On March 3rd, the healing process was getting better, but I had to have another surgery to fix my LP shunt valve... again. I hadn't even managed to go back to work from the previous surgery and I was faced with another.

At the end of March, we finally moved back to Bend. Coming home was exactly what we needed and Bend will always be our home. We got back to ourselves again and life became a little more fun. In April, Aaron and I went to a little farm with animals and a hot tub. There was also a dart board, but we kept on rooting our darts into the ground or the barn door. We always try to go away every month or so, if my health allows. We work hard, but there has to be a reason and a release. For us, that's making memories while we can.

Chapter Thirteen

May 2023 began with reminiscence and joy. A friend gave us a gift card to a fancy seafood restaurant called Anthony's. We went there for the sunset dinner and sat in a familiar booth, looking out the window at a familiar view. I suddenly remembered we had dinner there when Aaron worked in Bend a while ago. He didn't believe me until I pulled up photos of us in the same booth. Which one of us is the brain patient with no memory again?

On May 13th, my best friend Erika gave birth to my gorgeous little nephew Parker. I don't know if I'll live long enough to become an Auntie to my sisters' children but that little rugrat is like family so I consider him my nephew and spoil him accordingly. I met Erika in 2019 and we've been inseparable since. Aaron unknowingly got a package deal with us two. Amidst the absolute joy of Erika's latest arrival, something was going wrong. On May 17th, I had an MRI to check my shunts. They always have to be adjusted after an MRI, but instead of me traveling to Portland to get that done, the pharmaceutical rep kindly came to me. Aaron had always said that he wanted a shunt of his own.

I would reply, 'No, believe me, you don't.'

He would say 'I just want to see and touch one, that would be so cool.'

So, when the pharmaceutical rep arrived, he presented us with an LP shunt. Shunts have expiration dates and once expired they can't be used on humans, so vets use them for animals. Except that one was saved for us. Now it's our special little party trick where we can show people what's inside of me. It's all totally normal.

While waiting to find out what was happening with my shunts, we distracted ourselves with the baby trailer. As you know, we live in a trailer most of the time and love the freedom. We thought having a little trailer for small camping trips would be easier. Plus, when we didn't need it, we could rent it out. We found the perfect trailer, but it needed a lot of work. The couch and bed had been ripped out and it needed new floors and a few touch-ups. It was hard work but we had so much fun doing that project together and by the end of it, we had a lovely little trailer.

A week or two later, my Nana Nadia came to town. Aaron and I had our second-anniversary photoshoot booked for that week. Nana Nadia offered to drop us off and I suggested that she put some nice clothes on to come and meet our photographer friend Alesha. When we arrived, Nana Nadia was already right there so it wasn't too hard to convince her to join in with the photo shoot. We got some of the sweetest photos ever, and she and Aaron got some beautiful photos too. Nana Nadia adores my husband… I think she'd steal him if given the chance!

Later in June, we discovered that my VP shunt's valve was broken so I had to get a bunch of tests to ensure surgery was safe to go ahead. There was an MRSA test, a CBC, CMP, and PT/INR. They can't be too careful with VP shunt surgery because it can be incredibly dangerous. Once the tests came back clear, we began preparing. My friend started coming over to practice braiding my hair so they would only have to do minimal shaving. Once you've had no choice in shaving it off, hair feels much more important. They would have to reopen the scar that runs from the front to the back of my scalp, so she braided the hair away from that incision. All that practicing meant that she got it done very quickly on surgery day. When we were waiting for the date to come through, I was worried that it would end up happening on my birthday but thankfully, it was two days before. It would have been done sooner but Dr. D was on vacation and didn't want anyone else performing such an invasive surgery on me. It was my golden surgery; the 24th surgery within 24 years of life. It's not the sort of milestone you can find a celebration card for, but it's important to me. On July 12th, I had the VP shunt revision and ended up with six incisions. Three in my stomach and three around my neck and head. The typical person with IIH wouldn't need an incision on their neck for this surgery. However, they had to open me up to guide the tubing down into my chest because there was no excess fat or skin to push it through without causing extra damage. My neck and chest were badly bruised from the tubing being tunneled through and it took a while for that to heal. VP shunt surgery is often the worst recovery and it's always miserable. That's why I welcomed the trip to Aaron's family reunion a couple of weeks later. I had just had my sutures out so I was still struggling with the healing process and ended up secluding myself because of that. Regardless, it was nice to sit out in the sun. I switched between two hours of sunbathing and then two hours in bed repetitively for the whole four days. Aaron's family would sit in the shade, watching me bake in my special rocking chair, which is much less painful during recovery than an average chair. I'm always quite introverted at big family events so I enjoyed the peaceful company of the sunbeams. Although I did spend a lot of time chit-chatting about everything and nothing with my mother-in-law Gail, in between my sleeping and sunbathing.

On August 1st, we were home and decided to spend a week reno-
vating our trailer. Our kitchen wasn't the best, so we put in a huge new
sink and changed the countertop to a black marble effect with tones of
grey, gold, and brown mixed in. Aaron made it with epoxy and it looks
amazing. Life can be so fast-paced and stressful, but the DIY bubble
always gives us peace together. On August 4th, I finally went back to
work again and normality resumed once more.

That summer, Emilie was old enough to get her learner's permit
and when I visited my mom's house, she drove me everywhere. That
was terrifying. While we were out together, we went shopping and I
found a fancy black beret. I thought it was perfect for my and Aaron's
upcoming trip to Europe, but Emilie said it looked ridiculous. That
was rude. I brought Emilie back to Bend so she could spend some
of her summer with Aaron and I. While she was staying with us, I
mentioned that I had a Crumbl Cookie coupon in my purse with the
other 100 random coupons I had forgotten about.

Emilie and Aaron both turned to me with wide eyes and said,
'Crumbl Cookie? We have to go!'

I had no idea what all the fuss was about but when we got there, I
had a cookie that was overpriced and almost completely butter but it
was the best cookie I've ever had. After that, we took Emilie painting.
Us girls chose to paint canvases with such precision that the outcome
looked almost professional, whereas Aaron chose something different.
He made a tree, sunbeams, a shooting star, the moon, grass, and the sea
into one scene made of glass. Before it was melted, it looked amusing,
after it was melted, it looked hilarious. There's a photo of us all holding
our artwork and Aaron looks like a kindergartner smiling with the
macaroni art that he wants pinned up on the fridge. Before Emilie
went home, we also did an escape room where we had to be a tactical
response team trying to save a kidnapped girl from a bomb threat.

We're terrible at escape rooms but surprisingly, we got out with 1 minute and 24 seconds to spare. At one point, I played the dead guy and Emilie asked me to help by saying what I could see.

I replied, 'I see nothing, I'm dead!'.

It's funny how unimportant little things like cookies, jokes, and painting cause so much happiness in such a serious and uncertain life. It really is the little things.

In September, Aaron and I went ziplining with some friends in Mount Hood before it closed for the winter. It was incredibly cold up there, especially when the wind hit as we ziplined. One of the guys wore shorts and immediately regretted it. As we've established, I'm not supposed to go ziplining, but if I ever turn down the opportunity, you should be worried. A week or so later, my Nana Nadia ended up in hospital for a week. We never found out what was wrong, but the most concerning symptom was that she didn't recognize everyone. So, I took some time off work and visited her every day to comfort her and make sure there was a face that she knew. While I was there, I got interrupted by the monthly appointment in Eugene where I go to get injections in my neck and spine. I took that opportunity to make light of the hospital trip and take Emilie shopping before my upcoming trip to Rome. While our frequent trips make it seem like we live lavish lives, we don't. We work hard for these trips, which keep me going whenever life is all pain and appointments. I count the days until our next trip and put my focus on that.

In October, Aaron and I were supposed to travel to Rome before a cruise to the Holy Lands. I have always wanted to go because of how important my faith is to me. The day before we left for Rome, war broke out in Israel. We got notified that the cruise destinations had changed to Greece and Turkey. That was devastating news and I don't know if I'll live long enough to achieve that dream. Still, we were grateful for our safety and praying for those without that luxury. On October 10th, we flew to Rome. I kept checking for cheap upgrades and that night, I was offered an affordable upgrade to first class with fully reclining chairs. When they told us where to go for our connecting flight, Aaron thought there must be a mistake because we were economy, but I just shushed him and ushered him along until we got to first class. As we walked to our seats, he was like a puppy who just heard 'walkies'. I just accepted my free champagne as if I belonged there, but Aaron made no secret of his excitement. He kept showing me how the seats go up and down and up and down. One important piece of information: my husband snores. That night I had to constantly nudge him, shush him or tell him to roll over again because I could sense the first-class eye rolls.

Rome was a beautiful, one-of-a-kind trip. There were so many astounding cathedrals and monuments to see; we walked up to 15 miles a day to cram everything into our stay. One day, we walked up the Spanish steps and when we went to sit down we got whistled at by a policeman. We didn't know that you're not allowed to sit down on them. I understand why you can't, but, why would police yell at people for sitting on the historic site while ignoring littering on the historic site? The amount of litter in Rome was unexpected. I sent my mom a photo of it and she texted back, 'Are you in downtown Eugene?' Regardless, Rome was still astounding. One of my favorite places was the Pantheon Sundial. We got there when the sun was at its daily brightest and the way the beams shone into the dome was magical.

We traveled from Rome to Naples and Capri, then Kuşadası and Turkey, Cyrpus and then Piraeus, Santorini, Crete, Chania, and Rhodes in Greece. Finally, we returned to Italy before flying home.

That was one of my favorite cruises. The first day was an at-sea day and on the second, we went on the excursion to Pompeii. We saw the ancient chariot tracks in the stone road which the rain had filled. The houses were interesting, as the rich people had fancy mosaic floors yet the houses were all the same blueprints regardless of size. We went to a vineyard and farm where they demonstrated how to make mozzarella and afterwards, we were given some wine and cheese. The house wine tasted nasty and was very strong, as was the limoncello! I dipped my tongue in the limoncello and was immediately done with it.

The lady next to me said, 'I don't like it either, what do we do with it? They're about to hand out more!'

I swiftly placed every drop of that stuff in front of Aaron because he somehow enjoyed it. That day, we also visited Athens and did a guided selfie tour around the Colosseum, which was incredible. During that tour, we had a little trouble with the selfie stick and ended up with a reel of brilliant bloopers that were almost better than the proper photos. That evening when we boarded the cruise ship, we went to see a game show called Yes or No. Each contestant who went on stage had 2 minutes and 30 seconds to avoid saying 'yes' or 'no' otherwise they lost. Aaron told me to hit record so all our friends could see him win and then ran up to the stage with smug confidence. It took him exactly 20 seconds to say yes and he begged me to delete the video. I sent it to everyone we know.

On the ship, we met a lovely couple called Ivy and Joe, who people assumed were our parents so we jokingly called them mom and dad. On the fourth day, we visited Ephesus in Turkey. We went on a wine-tasting tour followed by a visit to a carpet shop where they would take people off to a dubious side room to sell the carpets. It seemed very shady, so when we were taken off with Ivy and Joe, we felt that playing along to annoy the sellers was simply the right thing to do.

I turned to Ivy with a pondering hand on my chin and said, 'Mom, I think this red one would look beautiful in your foyer.'

Eventually, we got bored of their persistence and had to argue that we weren't going to buy anything. Aaron and I escaped, whereas Joe and Ivy were practically held captive until they walked away while another couple bought a carpet. The tour guide made money on those sales, which is against the rules, and explains the shady set-up. I told her that it was immoral and then complained to the manager of the cruise ship who had no idea.

After that, we visited Greece. It was my job to plan the excursions and decide where we were going each day and I found somewhere called Pyrgos Kallistis. While everyone went on the planned excursion to Oia for the pretty painted houses and tourist hype, I got us a cab to Pyrgos. There were no crowds and nothing was pristinely painted or presented perfectly for tourists, which felt more authentic. What I loved was that everybody's houses were also little shops. So, we got to walk into people's lovely homes to see their unique, handmade items that no typical gift store would sell. There were also pieces of artwork hung up on the house's walls and they had little wooden shutters all painted sky blue. It was an eclectically beautiful village.

That evening, we went for dinner with two new friends at 'Chef's Table' which was the only restaurant run by the ship's head chef. They had a seven-course set menu... yes, seven. The woman that we were dining with had just turned 22, so we also had birthday cake on top of the seven courses. Each course was paired with a different wine and the world was spinning pretty fast by the night's end. They even gave us a bottle to take back to the room and asked us to not tell anyone but we instantly forgot that part. The chef had just got married at the last port and we got a photo with her in which I had no shoes on. We were all dressed up for the fancy restaurant, and as we walked in we looked fabulous but as we walked out, I was holding my heels and wobbling. The other woman and I ended up on the floor from laughing so hard while her boyfriend and Aaron tried to help us up. That was a great night.

The next day, despite probably having hangovers, we visited Chania on the Greek Island of Crete. As I was in charge, I googled 'things to do in Crete' and found the Old Town's colorful buildings and the historic Jewish Quarters. I wanted to go to a museum that sounded fascinating but as we arrived, we were greeted by a 'closed for today' sign. I was so annoyed but Aaron found it hilarious that they had been open for countless years and closed the day we arrived.

As we started to travel back around the map, we stopped for the final excursion day at Bodrum, Turkey. Aaron came down with a cold, so I went by myself to tour the magnificent Bodrum castle. I didn't stay alone for long because I met the sweetest old lady from our cruise there. We were walking up the castle stairs and they were triple the height of normal steps so that invaders would fall back down if they tried to run up them. The old lady was struggling with her walking stick so I helped her. It was hard enough for a young person! Together we looked through the holes that they used to shoot arrows through and learned that the side and back walls were thicker to protect the village from invaders' canons. I made another friend too- one with four paws and the cutest meow. My kitty companion followed me everywhere until the security guard wouldn't let him into the castle. That final evening on the cruise ship, the old lady bought Aaron and me drinks to say thank you. She said that she goes on so many cruises alone and nobody ever offers her help, which was sad to hear. That evening was the final fun activity of the trip: a salsa dancing class. When I looked back at the videos of myself dancing, I remembered the Kinesiology Tape. For years, I've had to use a brace or tape to keep my right kneecap in place while doing anything physical and I always used brown tape. When I was packing for Rome, I realized the brown tape would ruin my outfits so I found the pink tape and in all of the photos and videos from that trip, I have a fabulous bright pink knee.

At the end of the last day, I had a photo taken with my family of towel animals. Every time room service left a towel animal on our bed, I kept it and lined them all up on the couch. On the last day, I had accumulated a big family, including an alligator that held the TV remote in its mouth and an anteater who wore Aaron's sunglasses. My favorite part of that trip was the little village of Pyrgos, while Aaron's was Pompeii for its significance and Ephesus for the company of Joe and Ivy. We returned to Italy on October 23rd and flew home the next day. It was the perfect vacation and cleared my mind before making a big decision.

Chapter Fourteen

On November 3rd, after the idea had been suggested to me countless times by many people, I decided to start writing my story. If this book helps even one person with IIH feel understood or encourages someone with a chronic disease to make the most of life, then I have achieved my goal. I wanted to not only raise awareness of my condition but also show that despite being dealt difficult cards, you can still win. It might seem like I've included some small and insignificant memories, but every second of life is significant when you've surpassed your prognosis.

Another small memory from that week is when Aaron and I went bowling. Aaron is a great bowler, and when I lived in Wyoming I was too (because there was nothing else to do), but I left those skills in my teen years. In the first game, he bowled 230 and I bowled 144. In the second game, he got 164 and I got 50. So, we stopped before I embarrassed myself further. A few days later, I finally went to get myself checked out. During our vacation, I pushed through increasing pain in my head and neck but it kept getting worse, so I had no choice but to go to the hospital. They did abdominal X-rays to check my LP shunt for any leaks, but those showed no abnormalities. The doctors were once again stumped.

On November 16th, Aaron had to move to Pacific City for work but I couldn't join him because it was a six-hour drive from my work and appointments. So, Aaron took our trailer and I moved into a little cabin in Sunriver until he came back to set up the baby trailer for me. I much preferred the baby trailer because it was my own, and I got to decorate it with penguin Christmas decorations. However, I missed my husband and we had to spend Thanksgiving apart. I wasn't free to visit my family at that time either, so my boss kindly invited me over for Thanksgiving dinner and one of Aaron's colleagues invited me over the day after too. They both warmly welcomed me into their families for the day, which gave me extra reason to be thankful. After Thanksgiving, snow buried Sunriver and while Aaron was roasting by the beach, I was shivering in my trailer. I'm not the biggest fan of snow, which is ironic because I was raised in snow and I settled down where winter snow is commonplace. During those cold days, I came across a little brown tabby boy cat that looked identical to Boy Kitty. He kept coming to the trailer looking for warmth and food, so I looked after him as best I could until one day, he disappeared. I hope he found his owner if he had one. I adored having two of Boy Kitty for that short time.

On December 4th, I met up with a friend whose partner was also away for work, and we had a girly sleepover. We watched TV, chit-chatted, went over her wedding plans, and then she left super early for work the next morning. When I walked downstairs, I was greeted by an open front door and the realization that her huge dog was nowhere to be seen. I ran around the unknown neighborhood calling after a massive dog that I was slightly afraid of. Only recently a huge dog had run at me, so big dogs weren't in my good books- it solidified me being a cat person.

I found her wandering near a group of neighbors who asked, 'Is this your dog?'

I replied, 'Nope!' and dragged her away.

After that sleepover, I went back to the hospital for an MRI. I was still in more pain than usual and it was getting to a point where we needed to find out why.

At the end of December, Aaron and I both had time off for Christmas, so we rented a house near our families. On the first day of our stay, Emilie had a basketball cheer game. Her team won by two points in the last 12 seconds. Some kid amazingly shot the ball from half-court and made it. That team is ruthless and insanely good. They look like college kids already and they lose a maximum of one game per season. The next day, Erika and Parker visited, which was lovely. Parker is an incredible baby. He rarely cries and he smiles on cue, so we got gorgeous photos of him in his little Christmas outfit with a big toothless grin. In the few opportunities when everyone else was busy, my mom bombarded me with gifts because she bought me too many and didn't want me to open them in front of the others. They were 99% penguin-themed, which I loved. They included sneakers with so many penguins that they look like a *Where's Waldo* drawing, a penguin glasses holder, penguin flipper slippers, a red penguin scarf, and a penguin-shaped puzzle that still lays unsolved on my mother-in-law's table. We followed our usual traditions; on Christmas Eve we had dinner, opened gifts, and watched a movie at my mom's house. However, this time, we watched *A Charlie Brown Christmas* instead of *The Christmas Story*, which my mom always forces us to watch. We're big on traditions, as you can probably tell, and another is that we all bring one dish to dinner so that my mom doesn't have to cook everything. I always choose dessert because other than my mom, I'm the only baker. I usually make banana pudding, but it takes so long that I decided to make brownies instead. I wrote my name with the chocolate chips on top, so nobody asked who brought dessert. Emilie chose devilled eggs and she dyed them red and green to make them extra Christmassy. The dye pooled in the bottom, making them soggy and taste terrible. You couldn't pay us enough to eat them, but Steve took one for the team and ate a bunch of them.

During our traditional Secret Santa, my favorite gifts were the penguin called Regina from Emilie and the necklace that Aaron gave me. I have been gifted three adopted penguins over the years, all of which I could track. All three have been eaten by whales, including poor Regina. My penguins don't have the best of luck. The necklace from Aaron was very meaningful. While we were in Greece, I saw a silver necklace pendant of a little church and it was so beautiful but so expensive. I couldn't stop thinking about it and I regretted not buying it, so Aaron found the same one online and wrapped it up for Christmas. I wear it every day.

On the night of Christmas Eve, Aaron and I went to my mother-in-law's house and my parents joined us on Christmas Day for the prime rib dinner. My in-laws aren't gift-giving people so for once, I followed their ways and I didn't buy gifts for them. Except when I went by their rules, they went by mine and bought gifts for me! The next day, we went home and took Mercury to see Christmas lights- my favorite tradition.

Just as 2023 had ended, 2024 began- surrounded by family. My family came to Sunriver and ourselves, my parents, Emilie, Aunt Windi, my cousin Nicole, and niece Mia all stayed in one big house to celebrate Mom and Steve's anniversary. We spent a lovely couple of days shopping, eating, and laughing. However, on January 3rd, I started to feel worse. A slight fever started on the 5th and by the 8th, the pain was so bad in my head and back that I took myself to the ER. They admitted me and ran tests for two days. On the 10th, they discovered that my VP shunt was obstructed and I suspect that I had the start of an infection too (you'll soon understand why). I had surgery on the 12th and I was sent home on the 13th. A snowstorm raged outside and Portland was frantically being shut down as I recuperated in my hospital bed. My restless leg syndrome kicked in alongside the pain from the gas they used during surgery, so I needed to get up and walk. An uptight man called Dr. Adleton, who had been rude countless times in the past few days, saw me on my feet and said I was ready to go home. Nobody should go home one day after brain surgery, especially amidst a snowstorm, but I had no choice. Portland was blacked out and the hospital generators could only power the cardiology, neurology, and maternity wards. Later that day, they had to take power from the part of the neurology ward I had been in, so I was actually grateful to have been kicked out. Also, after I left, the pipes froze and burst, so they were evacuating people from dark, wet wards. When Aaron picked me up, I stepped out into an icy town in a state of panic. We come from the part of Oregon that isn't fazed by snowstorms, so we calmly decided to wait out the craziness in the hotel where Aaron was staying. When we arrived at the hotel, they had no power either so the elevator was down and the alternate route to the room was four flights of icy metal outdoor stairs. I could barely walk and Aaron began to panic, so I said I'd scoot up them on my butt if I had to. While Aaron took our stuff to the room, I waited in the freezing reception with the owner.

She asked, 'Are you staying because your house is bad from the storm?'

I replied, 'No, I just had my 25th brain surgery, that's all.'

She couldn't find an answer to that.

Eventually, Aaron helped me up the stairs on one side and a member of staff helped me on the other because the handrail was coated in ice. It took at least 20 minutes because I had to stop and rest after every few steps. We made it to our room and it felt like the Arctic. I doubled up on clothing layers and slid into bed to watch shows on my phone. Aaron went back out to find a second jump box so that we could use one to charge phones and one to jump-start the car in the morning. There was supposed to be a restaurant at the hotel but because the power was out, the staff went to the nearest store and bought sandwiches for everyone. Throughout the evening, I kept having to get up and walk the hallways because of the gas pain in my stomach and shoulders. The hallway was mostly unsheltered and faces peered through windows wondering why a shivering couple kept walking past at a tortoise's pace. The next morning, we went home. We drove on sheet ice for miles and passed at least six semi-trucks that got stuck or crashed. When we arrived in Sunriver, we got out of the car to find that the snow was up to my knees. It practically buried me- I'm only 5'2! Despite the weather, I was so glad to be home. I spent the next three weeks resting, reading, and playing *Red Dead Redemption*. I did nothing but hunt bears and Aaron kept telling me to play the missions, but following guidelines was no fun. Aaron was in between jobs, so for the first time, he was home for my entire recovery and I loved that quality time with him. Within those three weeks, the pain in my back and head vanished so I thought the issue was resolved. I always try to start easing myself back into normality after three weeks of recovery, so I gradually began doing things again. Over the next couple of weeks, the pain started to come back. When I returned to work and began lifting someone again, the pain in my back worsened. I thought it must be a herniated disc and the weeks of resting my back had kept the symptoms at bay for a while. So, I thought nothing of it.

At the end of February, Aaron was staying in Arizona for a week of training in his new job. I had four days between work shifts, so

I did my best to ignore my returning issues and flew to Arizona to meet him. He rented us a gorgeous red Corvette which I rode around town while he worked each day. One day I went to the Cerreta candy factory tour and made a chocolate teddy bear wearing a white sprinkled bikini for Aaron. They had a huge Santa mold that could hold 5000lbs of Chocolate and it had only been used once. I also visited the Historic Downtown Glendale District where all of the old houses have been made into shops. I went to the Spicery, Memory Lane, the Cottage Garden, and the Bears antique shop where I bought a 1930s newspaper with an advertisement for a $1000 cruise around Europe. There was also an *Alice in Wonderland*-style signpost with 'more shops' going in three different directions. In the evenings, Aaron and I explored together. One night we went to a restaurant called Flint where I had Swordfish. It was the meatiest, chewiest, most steak-like fish and I never intend to eat it again. We also went to a restaurant called The Compass which is almost entirely glass, very high up, and rotates, so that you get an amazing view of Arizona. The dark city looked beautiful all lit up with a million dazzling lights. My favorite evening in Arizona was when we visited Top Golf. I've been before and I'll admit that I'm terrible at it, but Aaron hadn't been before and I expected him to be better than me. Aaron shot his first ball and it flew upwards, bounced off the metal ceiling, and rained down on the very drunk party of six in the booth next to us. They ran around like headless chickens that thought the sky was falling. I suggested that he stop before someone died from a flying golf ball. My back and head pain was gradually increasing while I was there, but I didn't let it ruin our mini-trip. I flew home on February 29th to find more snow. I missed the warmth of Arizona already.

Once I settled in at home again, I called my doctors. Kareen also assumed it was a herniated disc, but she needed to order an MRI to check. If it was a herniated disc, I would have to get surgery again. I'm already on the muscle relaxants that they use to treat it and I already do physical therapy, which just leaves the option of surgery. However, my primary and secondary insurers suddenly decided that they had no idea who was primary so when Kareen asked for the MRI, nobody knew who should cover it and who should order it. Usually, the request is sent on week one, approved on week two, and done on week three. By week three, it still hadn't been approved. At this point, I couldn't stand upright without crying in pain. Aaron watched me get up from the couch and fall back down in agony. He told me to go to the ER, but I was stubborn. It's a four-and-a-half-hour drive to the Portland ER where my doctors are, so I wanted to make sure that it was bad enough to be taken seriously, or better yet, I wanted to wait for the MRI. On March 18th, I finally gave in and went to Portland. I had no idea that I would stay there for 25 days.

Chapter Fifteen

The week before I went to Portland, I decided I couldn't wait anymore, but I didn't want to go alone this time. So, I asked my mother-in-law Gail to come with me and we arranged to leave bright and early the following week. I barely managed to finish my work week, but I made it to Monday morning and met Gail at Portland ER. I explained my situation and as usual, I was considered a high priority because brain patients with shunts are always at a high risk of having a life-threatening issue. We waited two or three hours before they put me in a room and started me on Dilaudid, which is up to eight times stronger than regular morphine. I always need the strongest painkiller option because I have a very high tolerance due to being on daily fentanyl patches and oxycodone. Around 5 pm, they decided to admit me because I was in too much pain and needed tests which would have to be done the next day. I brought an overnight bag because I rarely get sent home, so that wasn't surprising. Gail stayed at a nearby hotel and the next morning, I woke up to coffee from Gail and normal X-ray results. The next step was the MRI that I had been waiting weeks for, but that came back normal too. Then they did a spinal tap. CSF is supposed to be translucent but mine was dark yellow. My opening pressure was 40, so combining those facts led to my CSF being tested and an infection being discovered. They brought my pressure down to 10 and started me on steroids, Vancomycin, Rocephin, and Ceftri-axone (that's a lot of antibiotics for one small human!). While there is no proof, I suspect that the infection started when my back and head pain began a few months ago. The pain was identical to then, just much worse. They started doing a spinal tap every 1-2 days to reduce the excess pressure. The first three IV lines that they put in all blew, so they decided to put in a PICC line which sent the antibiotics directly to my heart. It was uncomfortable at first but I didn't feel it after that day.

During my stay in January, I met a nurse called Abby who is the kindest, most dedicated nurse I have ever met. She made sure I never felt alone. I believe that all nurses deserve awards, but this one truly did, so I nominated her for a DAISY award. I saw her again in March and she showed me the plaque that she had won! I'm so glad she got the recognition she deserved, and I'm glad that she was there to keep me company this time too. I only saw Aaron on weekends due to work, so my mom and Gail rotated shifts at first. During the first few days, Dr. D said that he wanted to take out my shunts, put an outward LP drain into my spine (drains CSF into a bag), give me two weeks of antibiotics, replace the VP shunt, and then the LP shunt. Having an infection while having shunts is very dangerous and the doctors have to stop the infection from traveling to your brain at all costs. However, I showed no signs of a brain infection so my infectious disease doctor talked him out of it. We weren't sure what the new plan was but the antibiotics needed time to work their magic before anything else.

I started losing my vision on the 22nd of March. Each morning I looked at the grey and white clock on the wall opposite my bed but that morning, I couldn't see anything on the wall. They were doing spinal taps every day and my pressure was in the 20s and 30s, which was much lower than it had been so that didn't explain the vision loss. We had no idea what was happening, so I kept distracting myself in the few ways that I could. I went on walks up and down the corridors, I spent time with the hospital therapy dogs, I talked to whoever could visit me and if nobody could, the nurses made for good conversation. For the first two weeks of my stay, I wasn't allowed to go outside because of how high-risk my situation was. The infection, vision loss, and low blood pressure made the doctors worry that I would crash outside. My blood pressure has always been an issue (30/20 is my lowest and 50/40 is my highest!). Plus, I was having antibiotics put into my PICC line every hour, one after the other all day, so I couldn't wander off for long. I didn't realize that my vision loss was going to get worse or that I wouldn't be going home anytime soon, so everything still felt manageable. A couple of days later, we figured out that my LP shunt must be broken again. The valve on my VP shunt was still pumping so we had to assume that my LP shunt valve wasn't. The infection was also pinpointed to my lower back, where the pain had been for months, so the shunt was likely clogged in that spot. The new plan was the clear the infection and then fix the shunt.

On March 30th, I finally got to go outside for the first time and it was amazing. I was confined to a wheelchair and 30 minutes per day but it was better than nothing. After a few more days, they let me go outside for multiple 30-minute slots per day, as long as a visitor took me and I was back in time for the antibiotics. Then came Easter. My mom and Aunt Windi decorated my room with bright colors that I could see through my blurred haze and Aaron set up a doctor-themed photo booth with props to celebrate National Doctors Day. On April 2nd, Erika came to visit and we took doctor-themed photos, ate cafeteria food outside, and caught up with each other. There was a day when nobody could visit, so I was stuck inside, but the next day my mom was coming. I had a spinal tap that morning because I didn't feel the need for it the day before and my spine had one day off but that was the limit. Steve turned up instead of my mom and brought me a gift basket from my friend Ashley. We took our lunch outside but it started to rain on us, so I had another day of smelling disinfectant instead of flowers. I started to get a bunch more visitors and due to my mom's Facebook posts, I even got gifts from people all over the world!

The person that I wanted to see the most was Aaron, but I couldn't unless it was a weekend so I welcomed any company. My uncle Jim drove down from Northern Carolina, the little girl in the next room made beautiful drawings for me, and my friend Maria visited too. Maria works in a jail and she told me some of the juiciest jail stories that I could have happily lived without knowing. My friend Jamie and cousin Zac visited and they took me outside to eat pizza in the fresh air. Jamie had an app on her phone that identified flowers, so I asked her to tell me what each flower was and she used all her free tries so Zac downloaded it for me too. The flowers were the only interesting thing out there so I had to know them all, and then my 30 minutes was up. My mom brought Emilie to visit for a day, and she talked about her latest boyfriend so much that I made up a rule: 6 months of dating before I hear about him. That didn't work. After that, my boss' daughter and her children visited and brought the quilt which my boss handmade. It has purple roses, pretty patterns, bible verses, and a patch with my name on it. I loved that gift very much. I also remember that Joe and Ivy from our last cruise sent me adorable penguin cookies and one that said *I've had brain surgery, what's your excuse?* One of my most entertaining visitors was probably the harpist who plays for hospital patients. She played every song I asked for, including Fur Elise.

The hardest part about that entire pre-surgery ordeal was losing my vision. I remember in the first four days, Gail and I would look out of the big window in the corridor. The first time, I asked if she could see the train in the far distance and we bickered about this non-existent train for ages. Then, I saw a distant blue and white sign and asked if she could see the Walmart. We bickered again about the non-existent Walmart and for days after, we joked about it every time we went to the window. When I lost my vision, I stopped going to the windows. Instead, Gail would read my books to me. She would get into them so much that she twitched with anticipation as she turned the page. She even did an array of voices to go with each character, making listening much more enjoyable. When Jacob visited and I asked him to read, he spoke as if he was bored with the words coming out of his mouth.

I complained, 'Jacob, get into it! Be more alive!'

He replied, 'But these books are so stupid.'

I didn't much care for his incorrect opinion. He suggested audio-books but he sounded just like the robot that reads them. He also brought his Switch so we could play Monopoly. To roll the dice you could touch it or shake it gently and I hammered it back and forth until a nurse looked concerned and asked what I was doing.

I replied, 'Well, this is the only exercise I'm getting, I may as well make the most of it!'

When my mom visited, she didn't have time to play games or read because she would distract me in a million different ways. She would decorate my room, bring more visitors with her, get lunch with me, walk me around, and just talk for hours. Family and friends play an important role in keeping you sane when you're confined to the same four walls with no sight and no end to your stay in sight.

During that time, I had so many bags hanging onto my IV pole that the nurses called it my tree. The antibiotics were supposed to be one at a time, but I messed up the timing by being outside for too long, so I had multiple bags draining at once after that. I already knew how to start, stop, pause, and cancel IV antibiotics and I knew when the lines should be changed too. You pick up half of a nursing degree by being a permanent patient. My nighttime routine consisted of having antibiotics from 10 pm to 11 pm and then sleeping until the 7 am dose. One night, a new nurse came to administer the antibiotics. The machine started beeping and she couldn't figure out why. I said the lines needed changing but she replied that she had already done that. It was a bold move to claim she'd done it when I was watching her the entire time. By 11 pm, it was still beeping every minute or two and still no antibiotics. Then it was midnight and still no antibiotics. Abby finally came in and got it working...for ten minutes because the other nurse messed it up again. It was 2 am and thanks to this nurse, it was now beeping every 30 seconds. I was exhausted so I called Abby and begged her to let me go to sleep. In my opinion, sleep is equally as important as antibiotics and I wasn't getting either. She said that I could refuse this dose and continue in the morning, so I did. I also asked to never see that nurse again and thankfully I didn't.

Around that time, the doctors figured out that my vision loss was an incredibly rare allergic reaction to the steroids. It took about two weeks for my vision to fully return afterward, but it was quickly improving. Gail and I finally went back to the window to find Walmart.

On April 9th, I had surgery. They replaced all three components of my LP shunt (valve, catheter, and tubing) but they had to remove a lot of adhesions to make room for the new tubing. They always have to remove adhesions because the more surgeries you have, the more adhesions you get. They're making my stomach form as one because they combine and move organs until they're all in the wrong places. Dr. D hates doing LP surgeries on me because there's a high risk of him puncturing my organs when they pop up unexpectedly. I know that he can't predict where the organs are and I know the added risk, but tough, he has to keep going!

The recovery from this last surgery was easily the worst I've ever experienced. Maybe from the weeks of infection and antibiotics, maybe from the amount of adhesions removed- whatever the reason, I was more miserable and moody than ever. When Aaron tried to help me get comfortable, I shouted at him to not touch me. Once my pain meds were working, I apologized and he just laughed. He said it was like when a toddler has a tantrum and you probably should be mad at them but it's just funny. I didn't shout at him as badly as I thought I did, but it did make him understand that my pain was worse than ever. I couldn't lie down from the surgical gas pain and the incisions on my back and my front was hurting from more incisions. I was also still on antibiotics for the infection- those lasted for another few weeks. The whole ordeal was a lot for one body to go through. After 25 days, I finally got to leave the hospital. It was only a couple of days after surgery but on the 11th, I begged to go home. They wanted me to stay for at least three more days, but under the condition that I would come straight back if anything happened, they let me go. My mom drove me halfway home and I stayed with Aaron's parents for a few days. It broke up the long journey and it left me closer to the hospital, just in case. Aaron came to get me on his weekend off and I finally got to see my kitties, my husband, and my home again on April 14th. I absolutely couldn't have gotten through that past month without some great medical professionals, my wonderful family and friends, and the kindness and prayers from people across the globe. I'm grateful for the love that surrounds me and the miracles that have kept me on this earth until now. Life can be easily taken for granted, but when you've almost lost it countless times, you realize that it's a fragile, beautiful gift. Despite my battles, I'm still here to tell the tales and I thank God for that every day.

Chapter Sixteen

Conclusion

My past has been a difficult journey, my present continues to surprise me, and my future is as unknown as anybody's. Nobody's tomorrow is guaranteed. I was told to expect my last 'tomorrow' long ago, but I've won every risky poker game since. Every day I'm still here is a gift from God and I plan to make the most of his gifts.

Between my last surgery and finishing this book, Aaron and I have celebrated our third wedding anniversary and bought a five-and-a-half-acre property together. We love our trailers but decided it was time to build a permanent little home. I never thought I'd still be around to create a home of my own, but here we are. I will also have a she-shed, which will be filled to the brim with books, and Aaron will have a workshop. There are gorgeous mountains in front of the property and a blazing sunset behind it every night. Although Aaron always wanted to live in the city, we couldn't imagine living anywhere but the countryside now. In case I pass away before the house is built, Aaron has been told that he has to finish it and live in it for me. In these past few busy months, we have also visited a Renaissance Faire for Father's Day where we saw jousting, sword swallowing, and a fire act, I took Mercury on lots of car rides for pup cups, and I got a brain tattoo. I've always said I would never get a brain tattoo, but after twenty-six brain surgeries, I changed my mind. So, as an early birthday present from Aaron, I got a tattoo of my hands sewing my brain back together with a tiny '41' on the wrist. There's a quote that helped me to remember that in the Bible good things come after the suffering of forty, if you can just hold on until forty-one.

My plans for the rest of 2024 give me plenty to look forward to. I'll more than likely have more surgeries, but you can't plan life around uncertainties. We will be building our home for a while, and exactly one week from writing this, I will be turning twenty-six years old. I will be the same age as my amount of surgeries again and I will have surpassed my initial prognosis by one year. I have a birthday twin, Neia, who was born the same day and year as me (but I'm one hour older). Neia and I will celebrate with a girly weekend away getting pedicures, doing a photoshoot, and going bar-hopping. I've never been bar-hopping but she claims it's a rite of passage. From the end of September through to October, Aaron and I are going to London for a week then on a cruise to Spain, Portugal, and the Canary Islands. We're visiting a beer museum for Aaron in Spain, going on a tuk-tuk ride in Portugal, and riding camels in the Canary Islands. This year almost saw the end of me so I'm grateful to be here and making the most of the rest of it.

I have so many hopes for the future. I wish to see as much of the world as possible while I still can- that's always been very important to me. 2025 will hopefully include Bali, Greenland, or Iceland. I hope for fewer surgeries, but I will accept as many as God has planned for me. I hope to make countless more memories with my precious family and friends. I have hopes for each of those.

I hope that my little sister is always safe. She's growing up far too fast; she's sixteen this year. I hope that she lives a wonderful, happy, healthy, and safe life, even if I'm not here to watch over her. I hope that she marries the love of her life someday, has the beautiful life that she deserves, and lives every moment to the fullest. She's going to go so far in life, I just know it. I love you, Emmie.

I hope that my sister Olivia thrives doing whatever makes her happy for the rest of her life. I love you, Liv.

I hope that my mom will always be okay. She's been the most supportive, consistent part of this entire journey- holding my hand since day one. I pray that she and Steve remain happy and healthy for many decades more. I am beyond thankful for their devoted love and support. I love you, Mommy. I also hope that Steve keeps hunting and takes Emmie with him so that he always has a buddy- they need to keep that memory alive for me. I hope he knows that I've always loved him and he's taught me so much. Steve, I love you old man.

I hope that Jacob finds his soulmate and lives a full, content life. He's the perfect example of how a man should be. I hope he moves in with Aaron if they ever find each other alone. I love you, Brother.

Also, I hope that Zac always does whatever makes him happy, and keeps going to church on Sundays too. I love you, Zac.

I hope that my dad remains safe, happy, and loved. I love you, Dad.

I hope that Erika has a million more kids, just like she wants. I hope that her rugrats are taught about their Aunt Elise and hear all about the mischief that their mom and I got up to. I love you, Erika.

I hope that Mom and Dad Goetzinger live the longest, happiest lives. I know that they'll always be okay; they're some of the strongest people I know. I love you both.

I hope and pray that Aaron is always healthy and content. I hope that he builds our home, works in his shop, and if I can't, I hope that he finds someone else to look after him forever (but not too soon after me!). I hope that he has enough love and support to guide him through his grief someday. He deserves the longest, happiest, most travel-filled life. Sometimes he hates how much I make him travel but I hope he keeps doing it and sees the world for me. I hope that he keeps talking about me forever and never lets our glorious memories and dreams die. I couldn't love and appreciate him more...he's not one of the good ones, he's the best one. I would love nothing more than a lifetime with him. P.S. Aaron, don't put yourself in a mental institution like you always say you will after I go; I promise you'll be okay. I love you beyond words, Aaron James.

***

Every person on this earth fights a battle or two throughout their lives. Whether you are fighting a terminal illness, emotional challenges, or any of humanity's abundant struggles, you can overcome it. It may feel like you are breaking but know that you were given this battle because you are strong enough and you are not fighting alone. At the end of every difficult day, I remind myself that God gave me this fight because I am strong enough to handle it. If my story helps even one person to win their battle, that is the life I was destined to alter.

In the Bible, it rained for 40 days and 40 nights.
Day 41 came and the rain stopped.
Moses committed murder & hid in the desert for 40 years.
Year 41 came, and God called him to help rescue Israel.
Moses went up on the mountain for 40 days.
On day 41, he received the Ten Commandments.

Goliath taunted Israel for 40 days.

Day 41 came, and David slew him.

Jesus fasted and was tempted for 40 days.

Day 41, and the devil fled.

After His resurrection, Jesus appeared to His disciples for 40 days.

On day 41, He ascended into Heaven.

All this to say...don't quit. The rain will stop, the giant will fall, and you will enter your "promised land." Don't give up at 40.

41 is coming.' - McKenzie Miller

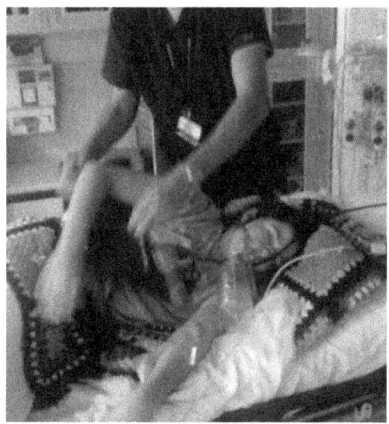

May 27th, 2013. After my life flight to Salt Lake City Primary Children's Hospital.

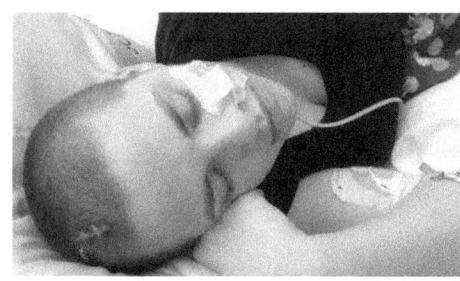

After my first brain surgery. I had a PICC line and an NG tube because according to the doctors, I was 'lifeless'.

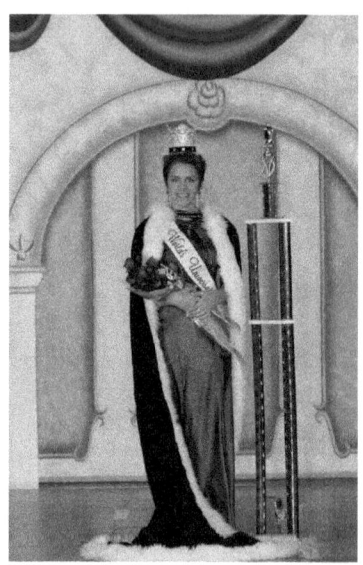

Beauty Pageant, 2015.

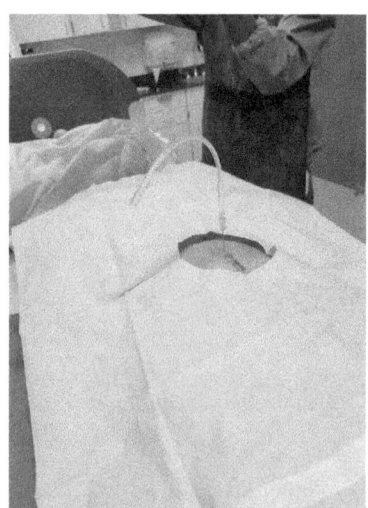

One of many spinal taps (lumbar punctures).

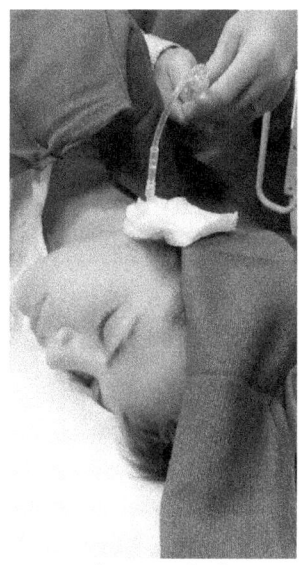

May 2nd, 2015. The shunt tap procedure which broke my VP shunt.

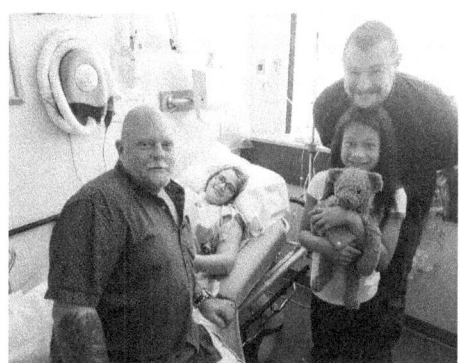

Surgery in June, 2018. From left to right: Steve (Stepdad), Me, Emilie, Aaron.

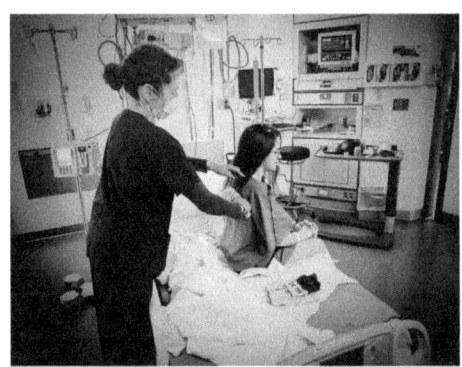

January, 2021: Chiari surgery. The nurse was brushing my hair.

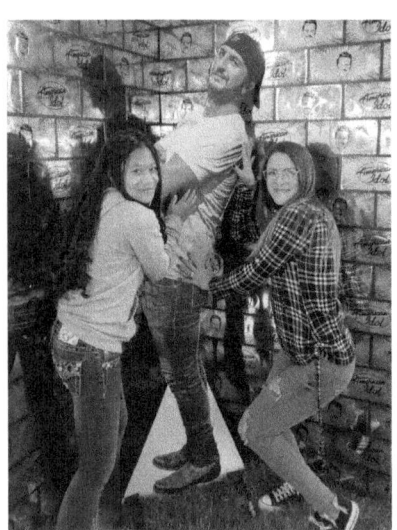

Luke Bryan concert in 2021 with Emilie (Sister).

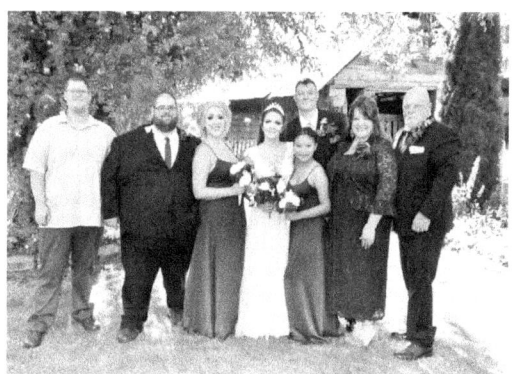

June 26th, 2021: Our wedding day. Left to right: Zac (Cousin), Jacob (Cousin), Olivia (sister), Me, Emilie, Aaron, Mom, Steve.

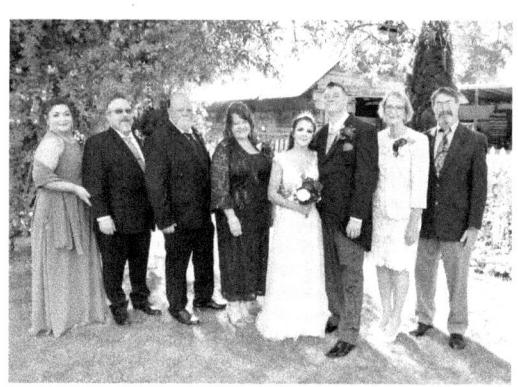

Our wedding day. Left to right: Pilar (Stepmom), Dad, Steve, Mom, Me, Aaron, Gail (Mother-in-law), Chuck (Father-in-law).

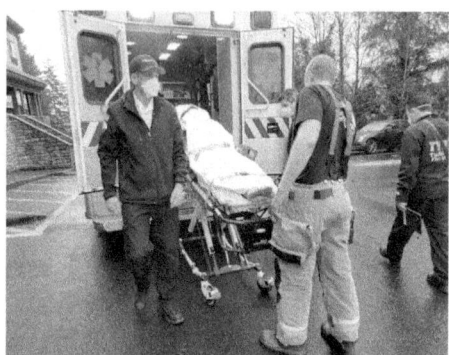

*January 19th, 2022. Ambulance ride from the
hotel back to the hospital after the 'simple'
surgery.*

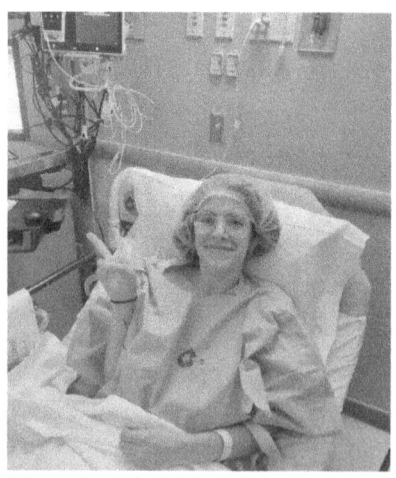

November 8th, 2022. CSF leak surgery.

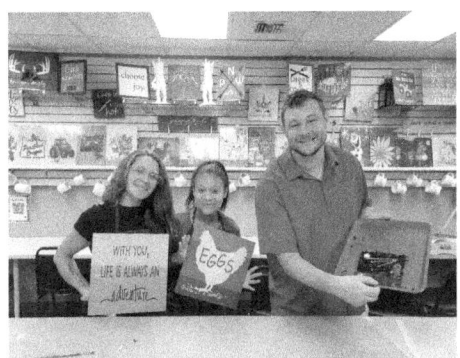

August, 2023. Left to right: Me, Emilie, Aaron.

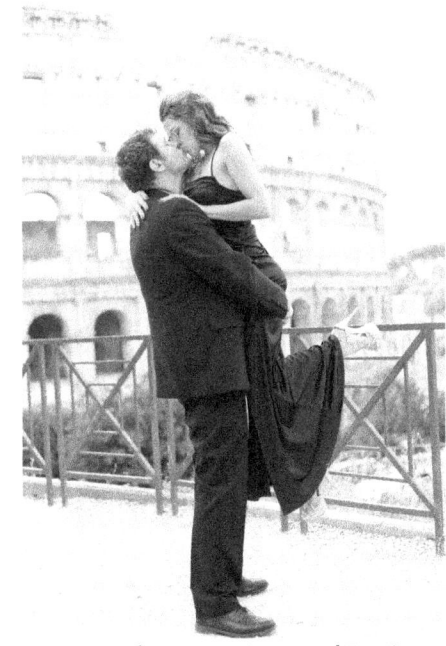

October, 2023. Aaron and I in Rome.

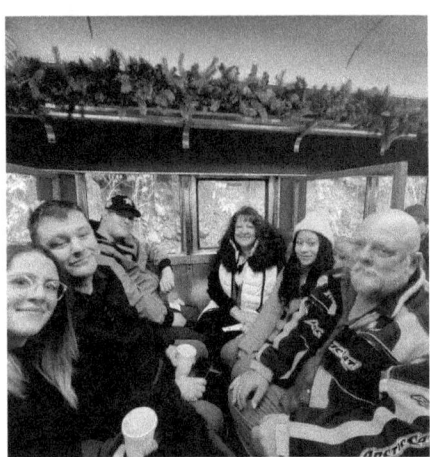

November, 2023. Left to right: Me, Aaron, Zac, Mom, Emilie, Steve.

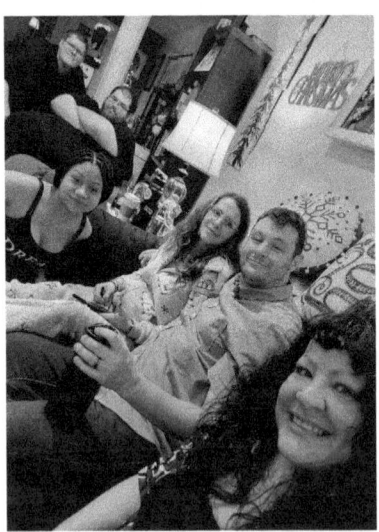

Christmas, 2023. Right to left: Mom, Aaron, Me (in penguin onesie), Emilie, Jacob, Zac.

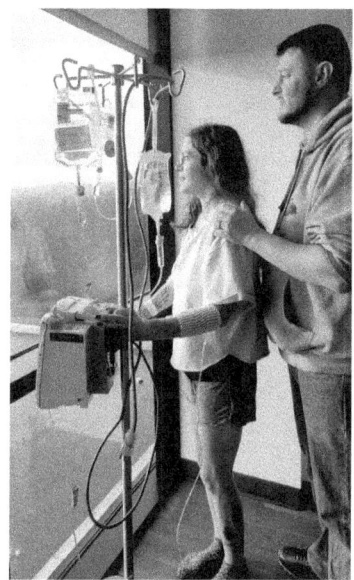

March-April 2024: 25 day hospital stay. Aaron and I looking out of the window, which I could not see out of.

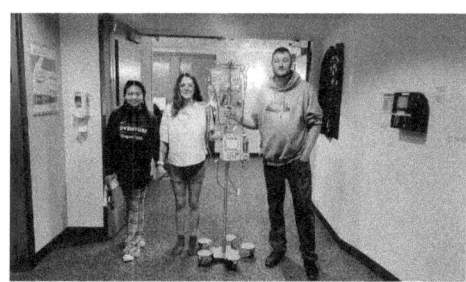

March-April, 2024: 25 day hospital stay. Left to right: Emilie, Me, Aaron.

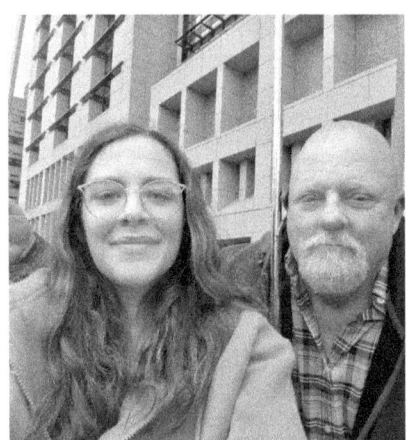

March-April, 2024: 25 day hospital stay.
Steve (Stepdad) and I.

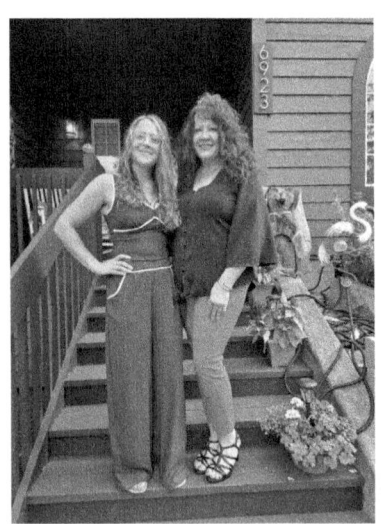

July, 2024. Mom and I.

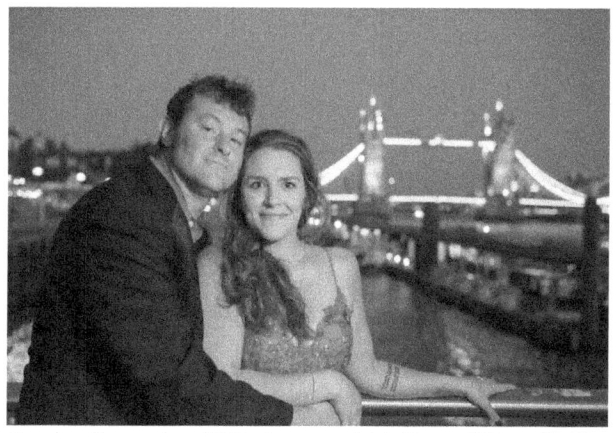

London: September, 2024. Aaron and I in front of Tower Bridge.

Please feel free to reach out to me on the following social media accounts:

counts:

Instagram: @egoetzinger21

Facebook: Elise Goetzinger

With special thanks to Tiffany for my book cover.

Cover art: Tiffany Rider

Instagram: @tiffanytattoos

For my husband and Mom who got me through countless battles, helped me through every step of creating this book, and will always have my heart.